third edition

MEDICAL TERMINOLOGY
Made Easy

Jean Tannis Dennerll, BS, CMA
Instructor/Coordinator of Medical Assistant and
Related Programs
Jackson Community College
Jackson, Michigan

Adapted from
**Medical Terminology:
A Programmed Systems Approach
8th Edition**

GENEVIEVE LOVE SMITH
PHYLLIS E. DAVIS
JEAN TANNIS DENNERLL

THOMSON

DELMAR LEARNING

Australia Canada Mexico Singapore Spain United Kingdom United States

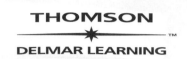

THOMSON
DELMAR LEARNING

Medical Terminology Made Easy, 3rd Edition
by Jean Tannis Dennerll

**Executive Director,
Health Care Business Unit:**
William Brottmiller

Executive Editor:
Cathy L. Esperti

Acquisitions Editor:
Sherry Gomoll

Development Editor:
Patricia A. Gaworecki

Editorial Assistant:
Jennifer Conklin

Executive Marketing Manager:
Dawn F. Gerrain

Channel Manager:
Jennifer McAvey

Project Editor:
Bryan Viggiani

Production Coordinator:
John Mickelbank

Art and Design Coordinator:
Connie Lundberg-Watkins

For permission to use material from this text or product, contact us by
Tel: (800) 730-2214
Fax: (800) 730-2215
www.thomsonrights.com

Library of Congress Cataloging-in-Publication Data
Dennerll, Jean Tannis.
   Medical terminology made easy / by Jean Tannis Dennerll.—3rd ed.
       p. cm.
   Includes index.
   ISBN 0-7668-2673-2 (alk. paper)
   1. Medicine—Terminology—Programmed instruction.
   I. Title.
   R123 .S6 2002
   610'.1'4'—dc21

                                    2002073719

NOTICE TO THE READER

The publisher does not warrant or guarantee any of the products described herein or perform any independent analysis in connection with any of the product information contained herein. The publisher does not assume, and expressly disclaims, any obligation to obtain and include information other than that provided to it by the manufacturer.

The reader is expressly warned to consider and adopt all safety precautions that might be indicated by the activities herein and to avoid all potential hazards. By following the instructions contained herein, the reader willingly assumes all risks in connection with such instructions.

The publisher makes no representation or warranties of any kind, including but not limited to the warranties of fitness for a particular purpose or merchantability, nor are any such representations implied with respect to the material set forth herein, and the publisher takes no responsibility with respect to such material. The publisher will not be liable for any special, consequential, or exemplary damages resulting, in whole or part, from the reader's use of, or reliance on, this material.

CONTENTS

LIST OF ANATOMIC ILLUSTRATIONS

The following rules are given as helpful guides:

"p" rule: A "p" at the beginning of a word followed by a consonant as in "pneumatic" and "psychology" is silent, but if the "p" is in the middle of a word and followed by a consonant as in "dysplasia," "dyspnea" and "eupnea" it is pronounced.

"g" rule 1: A "g " followed by **i, e, or y** is usually pronounced with a soft "g" sound like a "j" as in "giant, generate, or gymnast."

"g" rule 2: A "g" followed by an **a, o, u, or a consonant** is usually pronounced with a hard "g" sound as in "gate, got, gut, or ghost."

"g" rule 3: A "g" at the beginning of a word followed by the consonant "n" is silent as in "gnat," "gnaw," or "gnome." A "g" in the middle of a word followed by an "n" is pronounced like a hard "g" sound as in "ignore," "signature," or "diagnosis."

"c" rule 1: A "c" followed by **i, e, or y** is usually pronounced with a soft "c" sound like an "s" as in "city, cereal, or cycle."

"c" rule 2: A "c" followed by an **a, o, u, or a consonant** is usually pronounced with a hard "c" sound like "k" as in "cast, code, cut, or truck" (exception, "ch" like "church").

PREFACE

Medical Terminology Made Easy, **3rd edition**, is the book for you. If you are a student entering a health career program, such as medical assisting, or returning to a medical career after an extended absence, a volunteer for the Red Cross or a Hospice, a health information technician or manager, a health unit coordinator, nursing assistant, public health record keeper, aspiring medical transcriptionist, court reporter or legal assistant, medical insurance biller or claims adjuster, attorney, medical administrator, environmental control technician, social worker, educator designing short or noncredit courses, or an individual seeking personal knowledge, *Medical Terminology Made Easy,* **3rd edition**, is designed to meet your needs.

This programmed-learning, self-paced text is designed to ease you into the language of medicine that separates the layperson from the professional. The following features assist you in your goal of being able to pronounce, spell, define, and build medical terms.

Ten units are grouped by topic and body system, and **programmed learning** is perfect for learning a word-building system. It introduces prefixes, combining forms, and suffixes. You will soon be correctly defining and building hundreds of medical terms.

New and revised review exercises are included at the end of each unit. Divide and Define, Matching, Word Building, Sentence Completion, and labeling diagrams have been written to increase interaction with terms and enhance learning.

New crossword puzzles have been written and may be found at the end of each unit.

Abbreviation lists that relate to **each unit** and an abbreviation self-test follow each unit. A complete list of abbreviations, including weights and measures, chemical symbols, diagnoses, procedures, and charting abbreviations, is located in **Appendix A**.

Color illustrations with structures that have been labeled with names and combining forms appear throughout the text.

A pronunciation key is placed at the beginning of the text, including rules and **phonetic spellings** that appear below the term listed in the answer column. All of the pronunciations have been reviewed using *Taber's Encyclopedic Dictionary*, 19th edition (F. A. Davis), *Dorland's Illustrated Medical Dictionary*, 28th edition (Saunders), and *Stedman's Medical Dictionary*, 27th edition (Lippincott, Williams, & Wilkins) as references.

Several new appendices have been added:

Appendix A continues to list medical abbreviations.

Appendix B contains a comprehensive history and physical exam report.

Appendix C presents a new list of proper noun medical terms that do not easily fall into the word-building system.

Appendix D is a list of additional word parts not taught in the units.

Appendix E includes answers to review exercises.

Appendix F gives crossword puzzle solutions for each unit.

Special frames called **Spell Check** and **Career Profile** have been written to focus the learner on troublesome spelling concerns and to feature various types of medical practitioners.

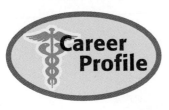

An audio CD-Rom is included with the text. It reviews the most important terms and gives the definition and a final pronunciation. This is especially useful to practice pronunciation, to copy as dictation, and check spelling, or to listen to in the car, around the house, or on the computer for extra study time.

An instructor's manual, with sample syllabi, class organization, games, quizzes, midterm and final exams, and additional case studies, may be ordered through your Delmar representative.

As you will see, *Medical Terminology Made Easy*, 3rd edition, is intended to provide you with a tool for self-directed learning that makes the study of medical terminology a practical, interesting, and pleasant experience. Your comments are welcome, and we hope you enjoy this new edition.

Jean Tannis Dennerll, BS, CMA

ACKNOWLEDGMENTS

This new edition would not be possible without the dedicated professional team at Delmar Learning, including: Sherry Gomoll, Patty Gaworecki, John Mickelbank, Bryan Viggiani, Connie Lundberg–Watkins, and Jen Conklin.

Many expert reviewers also contributed their valued opinions. They include:

Rachel Allstatter, LPN, BSEd, MED, CMA
Southern Ohio College
Cincinnati, OH

Pamela A. Eugene, BAS, RT (R)
Assistant Professor
Allied Health Division
Delgado Community College
New Orleans, LA

Mary Chiaravalloti, RN, CMA
Bryant & Stratton College
Buffalo, NY

Linda Curda, BS, MPH
University of Alaska
Bethel, AK

Jane A. Hlopko, MA, RHIA
Associate Professor
Broome Community College
Binghamton, NY

Fred R. Pearson, Ph.D.
Professor of Public Health
Brigham Young University Idaho
Rexburg, ID

Sally Pestana, MT (ASCP)
University of Hawaii
Honolulu, HI

ACKNOWLEDGMENTS

Diane Rider, RN
Lake Area Multidistrict Center
Water Town, SD

Janice Walbert, BA, REEG/EPT
Director
School of Electroneurodiagnostics
St. John's Hospital
Springfield, IL

Mary Walker, AS, BS, ART, CMT
Southwestern Technical College
Jackson, MN

Mary E. McGillivray Walker, M.Ed., RHIA, CCS, CMT
Instructor
Minnesota West Community and Technical College
Jackson, MI

My continued love and gratitude go out to my husband, Timothy, children, Diane and Raymond, and my mother, Helen Tannis, for their support in my work.

In Memoriam:

Medical Terminology Made Easy, 3rd edition, is specially dedicated to Noreen A. Calus, MS, RRA, a health information management administrator and educator who passed away in 2001. Ms. Calus provided expert and dedicated research on review of the medical terms in this text and remained a credentialed member of the American Health Information Management Association despite her battle with multiple sclerosis. We are grateful for her contribution to this text.

ABOUT THE AUTHOR

Jean Tannis Dennerll, BS, CMA, is a graduate of Eastern Michigan University. She earned degrees in biology, psychology, and education. She attended graduate school at Michigan State University and has completed many hours of continuing education, as well as presenting as a speaker at the AAMA, AAMT, MSMA, and other professional workshops. Ms. Dennerll became a certified medical assistant in 1979 and continues to be active on the local, state, and national levels of the American Association of Medical Assistants, as well as participating in Michigan Medical Assistant Post-Secondary Educators (M-MAPSE). For over 25 years she has been the instructor and coordinator for the medical assistant, unit coordinator (clerk), medical billing, and medical transcriptionist programs at Jackson Community College, and is coauthor with Genevieve L. Smith and Phyllis E. Davis of *Medical Terminology: A Programmed Systems Approach*, 8th edition (Delmar Publishers, 1999). Ms. Dennerll is married to Timothy J. Dennerll, Ph.D., has two teenage children, and lives in Jackson, Michigan.

How You Work the Program

1

frame

Now go on to Frame 2

DIRECTIONS: Cover the answer column with the marker provided as part of the back cover. A frame is a piece of information, plus a blank (_____)in which you write. All this material following the number 1 is a _____.
Check your answer by sliding down your cover paper.

2

correct

Now go on to Frame 3

By checking your answer immediately, you know whether or not you are correct. This immediate knowledge helps you learn only what is _____ (correct/incorrect).
Check your answer by sliding down your cover paper.

3

write

Writing your answer in the blank or on a separate piece of paper aids learning. Use the blank or a separate paper
to _____ your answer.

4

program

Programmed learning is a way of learning that gives you immediate feedback and allows you to work at your own speed. When you work a series of frames and are certain that you know the terms, you are learning through a
_____.
Check your answer by sliding down your cover paper.

5

check

write

Always _____ your answers immediately.
Always _____ your answers in the blank or on a separate paper.

ANSWER COLUMN

6

When you see _____ (a blank space), your answer will need only one word. In the sentence, "This is a program in _____ terminology," you know to use _____ word.

medical
one

7

Whenever you see an asterisk and a blank, *_____, your answer will require more than one word. In the sentence, "This is a programmed course in *_____," your answer requires *_____.

medical terminology
more than one word

8

In *_____, there is no clue to the length of the words. The important thing to remember is that *_____ means *_____.

more than one word

9

When you see a double asterisk and a blank, **_____, use your own words. In the sentence, "I think a programmed course in medical terminology will be **_____," you are expected

**_____.

anything from
  interesting to dull
  (if you did not
  answer this one, it
  doesn't matter)
  use your own words to

10

In the sentence, "I want to go to college because **_____," you are free to **_____.

use your own words

ANSWER COLUMN

11

Do not be ashamed of a mistake; this is not a test. If you make an error, simply look _____ to see where you were incorrect, then _____ the error.

back
correct

12

Summarize what you have learned about the mechanics of working a program:

_____ means _____ word.
*_____ means *_____ word.
**_____ means **_____ words.

one
more than one
use your own

13

Continue to summarize:
Any error must be *_____.
You may always look _____.
Never look _____.
This is not a test. It is a way of _____.
Use the blanks to _____ your answer.
Always check your _____ with the column on the left.

corrected in writing
back
ahead
learning
write
answer

14

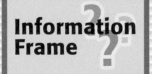

Information Frame

The material to be learned in the first frames is the most important part of the entire course. This teaches the **system** of word building you will use in *Medical Terminology Made Easy*.

15

Medical dictionary

This program requires the use of a medical dictionary.
Keep one handy and look up each new term as you learn it. Notice that the dictionary will give information on word origins, definitions, pronunciation, and usage.

The Word-Building System

16

Medicine has a large vocabulary, but you can learn much of it by word building. When you put words together from their parts, you are _____ building.

word

17

All words have a word root. Even ordinary, everyday words have a *_____.

word root

18

The word root is the foundation of a word. Trans/**port**, ex/**port**, im/**port**, and sup/**port** have **port** as their *_____.

word root

19

Suf/**fix**, pre/**fix**, af/**fix**, and **fix**/ation have **fix** as their *_____.

word root

20

The word root for tonsil in **tonsill**/itis, **tonsill**/ectomy, and **tonsill**/ar is _____.

tonsill

21

Look up the word tonsillitis in your medical dictionary. What language is the word root from? _____ Write the definition here: *_____.

Do it!

ANSWER COLUMN

22

Compound words can be formed when two or more word roots are used to build the word. Even in ordinary English, two or more word roots are used to form

compound words

*_____ as in "highchair," "firefighter," and "grandparent."

23

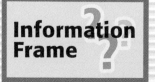

A slash mark "/" is used to divide words into their word parts.
Example:

gastr/	o/	duoden/	o/	stomy
word root/	combining vowel/	word root/	combining vowel/	suffix

24

A **combining form** is a **word root** plus a **vowel**.
In the word therm/o/meter, therm/o is the

combining form

*_____.

25

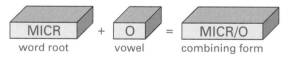

MICR (word root) + O (vowel) = MICR/O (combining form)

micr is a word root meaning small.

combining form

micr/o is the *_____.

26

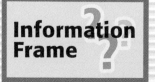

Adding a **vowel** (a, e, i, o, u, or y) to a word root to create a combining form allows two or more word roots to be joined to form a **compound word**. It also allows a word root to be joined with a suffix to form a word. In addition, the vowel assists by making the term easier to pronounce.

ANSWER COLUMN

vowel, "o"

27

In the word speed/o/meter, the *_____
allows "speed" to be joined to "meter."

combining form

28

In the words micr/o/scope, micr/o/film, and micr/o/be,
micr/o is the *_____.

compound words

29

Because they are formed by joining two or more word roots,
therm/o/meter, speed/o/meter, micr/o/scope, and
micr/o/film are all *_____.

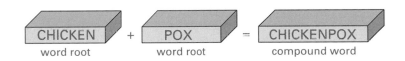

CHICKEN + POX = CHICKENPOX
word root   word root   compound word

Information Frame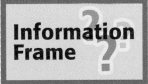

30

Use a combining form when joining a word root to a suffix or
another word root that begins with a **consonant**.
Examples:
1. gastr/o/duoden/o/scopy

combining form	**combining form**	**suffix**
gastr/o	duoden/o	scopy

2. micr/o/scope

combining form	**word root (suffix)**
micr/o	scope

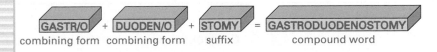

GASTR/O + DUODEN/O + STOMY = GASTRODUODENOSTOMY
combining form combining form suffix compound word

ANSWER COLUMN

would

neur/o/spasm

31

You (choose one) **would/would not** use a combining form to join the following word roots: "neur" and "spasm" to form _____.

32

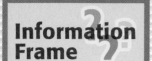

It is usually not necessary to use a combining form when joining a word root with a suffix or another word root that begins with a **vowel. Examples:**

1. **dermat/itis**

word root   **suffix**
dermat   itis

2. **hidr/aden/itis**

word root   **word root**   **suffix**
hidr/   aden/   itis

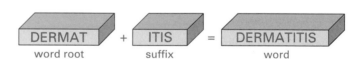

33

would not

lymph/adenopathy

You (choose one) **would/would not** use a combining form to join "lymph" and "adenopathy" to form _____.

NOTE: Combining forms are never used as an ending. They require an ending to complete a word. There are many exceptions to the rules about combining form usage, stated above. Always consult your medical dictionary for correct spelling of new terms.

34

combining form
word

Compound words can also be formed from a **combining form** and a **whole word**. Thermometer is a compound word built from a combining form and a word. In the word therm/o/meter:
therm/o is the *_____ ;
meter is the _____.

ANSWER COLUMN

35

Build a compound word from the combining form **micr/o** plus:

micr/o/scope   scope micr /o/_____.

micr/o/film   film   micr /o/_____.

micro/o/meter   meter micr /o/_____.

36

In medical terminology, compound words are usually built from a **combining form**, a **word root**, and an **(ending suffix)**. In the word micr/o/scop/ic:

micr/o is the combining form,

scop is the word root,

ending (suffix)   ic is the_____.

37

In the word son/o/graph/ic:

son/o is the combining form

word root   **graph** is the *_____,

ending (suffix)   ic is the _____.

38

In the word acr/o/megal/y:

combining form   acr/o is the *_____,

word root   megal is the *_____,

ending (suffix)   y is the _____.

39

Build a word from:

the combining form hydr/o,

the word root   chlor,

the ending   ic.

hydr/o/chlor/ic   _____

hī drō **klor'** ik

ANSWER COLUMN

40

Build a word from:
the combining form hydr/o,
the word root   chlor,
the ending   ide.

_____ (HCl)

hydr/o/chlor/īde
hī drō **klor'** id

41

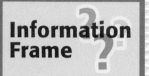

Information Frame

If you are unsure of the last two frames, rework the program starting with **Frame 36**.
NOTE: The last part of the word usually appears first in the definition, i.e., inflammation (itis) of the bladder (cyst)—cystitis.

42

The ending that follows a word root is a suffix. You can change the meaning of a word by putting another part after it. This other part is also called a _____.

suffix

43

The suffix er means **one who** or **one which**. The word root, port (to carry), is changed by putting er after it. In the word port/er, er is a _____ meaning one who carries.

suffix

44

one who

A medical practitioner is *_____.
practices medicine.

45

In the word read/able, able changes the meaning of read.
able is a _____.
Study the following table of noun and adjective suffixes, their meanings, and examples.

suffix

Noun Suffixes	Medical Examples
ism—condition, state, or theory	hyperthyroidism
tion—condition or action	contraction
	relaxation
ist ⎫	psychiatrist
er ⎭ —one who	practitioner
ity—quality	sensitivity

Adjectival Suffixes	
ous—condition, material	mucous
	nervous
able ⎫	inflatable
ible ⎭ —ability	edible

46

Now that you have studied the table of suffixes, use what you have learned to build a word that means:
able to flex _____;
quality of being active _____;
state of being contaminated _____;
one who creates sonograms _____.
Good job!

flex/ible
activ/ity
contamina/tion
son/o/graph/er

ANSWER COLUMN

47

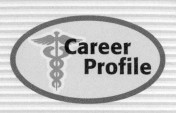

Nurses: LPN, RN, nurse anesthetists (CRNA), and nurse practitioners provide routine-to-complex nursing care for patients in acute and ambulatory care facilities. The scope of practice for each nurse is determined by the level of education and type of licensure from certificate programs to Ph.D.s.

48

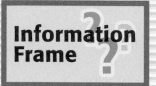

Suffixes also may change the part of speech of a word. For example, nouns (naming persons, places, or things) may be changed to adjectives (descriptors) such as:

Noun	Adjective
cyan/osis	cyan/otic
anem/ia	anem/ic
muc/us	muc/ous
ili/um	ili/ac
condyl/e	condyl/ar
carp/us	carp/al

49

osis

ia, um

In the words cyan/osis, anem/ia, and duoden/um, the noun suffixes are _____, _____, and _____.

50

ac

tic

ic

al

ous

ar

List the suffixes that make the following nouns adjectives:

Noun	Adjective
ilium	ili/ac
cyanosis	cyan/o/tic
anemia	anem/ic
duodenum	duoden/al
mucus	muc/ous
condyle	condyl/ar

ANSWER COLUMN

Information Frame

51

Verbs are words that represent action or a state of being.
Examples: incise, ambulate, love.

52

The suffixes -ed or -ing added to the verb **plant** alter the tense of this verb (when the action takes place). Create the past tense by adding "ed" to plant:

planted

_____, and the present participle by adding "-ing" to plant:

planting

_____.

53

The word part that follows a word root is a

suffix

_____.

54

adjective
verb

A suffix may change a noun to an _____ or change the tense of a _____.

55

Prefixes are word parts that are placed at the beginning of a word or in front of a word root to change its meaning. Recall from Frame 18 that trans/port, ex/port, and sup/port are all built from the word root port, meaning carry. Trans-, ex-, im-, and sup- are prefixes that alter the meaning of "port." Look these words up in your dictionary and write the meanings you discover for the following prefixes.

across or over
removal or out from
in, bring in, or not
up from under or hold up

trans-_____
ex-_____
im-_____
sup-_____

ANSWER COLUMN

56

Thinking exercise

Think of the meaning of the prefixes as you read these medical terms and their definitions:

trans/derm/al   across or through the skin (adjective)
ex/pir/ation   breathing out (condition)
im/plant   to place inside

Prefixes are an important building block in medical terms, and you will learn many as you progress through your studies.

57

Now for a review of the Word-Building System. Complete the following statements:

word root

The base of a word is the *_____.

vowel

A combining form is a word root plus a _____.

Two or more word roots or combining forms used to build a word

compound

make up a _____ word.

The word part that is placed at the end of a word to change its

suffix

meaning or part of speech is a _____.

prefix

A _____ is placed at the front of a word to change its meaning.

Notice the diagrammed sentence below, which illustrates the use of adjectives, nouns, and verbs.

```
        adj      noun    verb        adj     noun      adj     noun
The medical assistant charted the patient's history of duodenal ulcer.
   └──────────────┬──────────┘   └──────────────────┬──────────────────┘
              subject                            predicate
```

Notice the diagrammed words below indicating their word parts:

dysmenorrhea

dys	men	o	rrhea
prefix	word root		suffix
	combining form (vowel)		

acrodermatitis

acr	o	derma	itis
word root		word root	suffix
combining form (vowel)			

PRONUNCIATION NOTES:
Pronunciation symbols, descriptions, and rules are described on the inside front cover. They will also appear throughout the text below new terms and at other appropriate times. Refer to this pronunciation key or your medical dictionary when in doubt about how to say a word.

How do you know what to put where? In the following pages, you will find material to assist you with word building. This is a system that you may have already figured out. If not, study these rules.

RULE 1:
Usually, the definitions indicate the last part of the word first. The descriptive phrases usually start with the suffix and then indicate the body part.

Examples

1. Inflammation of the bladder
   inflammation   /itis
   (of the) bladder   cyst/
                      cyst/itis

2. One who specializes in skin disorders
   one who specializes (studies)   / /logist
   (in) skin (disorders)   dermat/o/
                      dermat/o/logist

3. Pertaining to the abdomen and bladder
   pertaining to   / / /ic
   (the) abdomen   abdomin/o/ /
   (and) bladder   / /cyst/
                   abdomin/o/cyst/ic

RULE 2:
Where body systems are involved, words are usually built in the order that organs are studied in the system.

Examples

1. Inflammation of the stomach and small intestine
   inflammation   / / /itis
   (of the) stomach   gastr/o/ /
   (and) small intestine   / /enter/
                    gastr/o/enter/itis

2. Removal of the uterus, fallopian tubes, and ovaries
   removal of   ____ / / ____ / / ____ /ectomy
   (the)uterus   hyster/o/ ____ / / /____
   fallopian tubes   ____ / /salping/o/ ____ /____
   (and) ovaries   ____ / / ____ / /-oophor/____
                      hyster/o/salping/o/-oophor/ectomy

   Of course, prefixes still come in front of the word.

Guide for Plural Formation

Since most medical terms are taken from Greek and Latin, they use the rules from those languages to form plurals. In English, we usually just add an "s" or an "es" to a word to make it plural, but there are many other possibilities used in medical terminology. The following will help you in medical terminology plural formation:

Singular Noun Ending		Plural Noun Ending	
a	(vertebra)	ae	(vertebrae)
us	(bronchus)	i	(bronchi)
um	(atrium)	a	(atria)
ma	(carcinoma)	mata	(carcinomata)
on	(spermatozoon)	a	(spermatozoa)
is	(pubis)	es	(pubes)
ix	(cervix)	ices	(cervices)
ex	(apex)	ices	(apices)
ax	(thorax)	aces	(thoraces)

As you look up terms in your dictionary, check the plural form mentioned with the pronunciation and the definition. You are now ready to begin Unit 1.

WORD-BUILDING SYSTEM REVIEW ACTIVITIES

Circle the correct answer.

1. The base of a word is its _____.

   a. combining form　　　　　b. adjective
   c. word root　　　　　　　　d. plural form

2. A word root plus a vowel is a(an) _____.

   a. noun form　　　　　　　　b. adjective form
   c. word root　　　　　　　　d. combining form

3. A word built from two or more word roots is a(an) _____.

   a. compound word　　　　　b. adjective
   c. plural　　　　　　　　　　d. combining word

4. A suffix may be used to do all except:

   a. Change the part of speech of a word
   b. Change the meaning of the word
   c. Change a singular to a plural
   d. Join two word roots together

5. Which of the following suffixes indicates a person?

   a. -ous　　　　　　　　　　b. -able
   c. -osis　　　　　　　　　　d. -er

6. The suffix -ism indicates a(an):

   a. verb ending　　　　　　　b. adjective ending
   c. condition　　　　　　　　d. inflammation

7. Which of the following is not an adjective?

   a. anemic　　　　　　　　　b. cyanosis
   c. carpal　　　　　　　　　d. mucous

8. Which of the following is the correct use of a combining form?

   a. hydrchloride　　　　　　b. chickenopox
   c. dermatoitis　　　　　　　d. microscope

9. Words that show action or state of being are called:

   a. verbs　　　　　　　　　　b. nouns
   c. adjectives　　　　　　　　d. prefixes

10. Names of body parts and diseases would most likely be _____.

    a. verbs　　　　　　　　　b. nouns
    c. adjectives　　　　　　　d. plural

ANSWER COLUMN

Practicing Plurals: Form the correct plural from the following singular terms:

1. bacillus _____

2. diagnosis _____

3. cervix _____

4. ganglion _____

5. ilium _____

6. lipoma _____

Transforming Nouns to Adjectives: Form the correct adjective from each of the following nouns:

1. cyanosis _____

2. anemia _____

3. carpus _____

4. ilium _____

Now, check your answers in Appendix E.

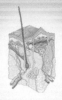

UNIT 1
Introduction to Medical and Anatomical Terminology

Study these word parts, meanings, and examples. Then proceed to the first frame.

WORD ROOT/COMBINING FORMS
abdomin/o (abdomen)
acr/o (extremities)
anatom/o (body structures)
anter/o (front)
blast/o (immature/embryonic cell)
caud/o (tail)
cephal/o (head)
cyan/o (blue)
cyt/o (cell)
dermat/o, derm/o (skin)
dist/o (distant from origin)
dors/o (back)
epitheli/o (epithelial)
eti/o (cause of disease)
hist/o (tissue)
later/o (side)
leuk/o (white)
medi/o (middle)
megal/o (enlarged)
muc/o (mucus)
pelv/o (pelvis)
physi/o (function)
pleur/o (lung cavity)
poster/o (back)
proxim/o (closer to the origin)

ser/o (serum or serous membrane)
thorac/o (chest)
ventr/o (front)

SUFFIXES
-centesis (surgical puncture)
-cyte (cell)
-ia (condition)
-ist (a person who)
-itis (inflammation)
-logist (one who studies)
-logy (the study of)
-megaly (enlarged)
-meter (instrument to measure)
-metry (process of measuring)
-osis (condition or increased number)
-paralysis (loss of movement and feeling)
-pathy (disease)
-tic, -ous, -ic, -al (adjective endings)
-um, -y, -a, -us (noun endings)

Word Examples

WORD ROOT/COMBINING FORMS

abdominal
acromegaly
anatomy
anterior
blastocyte
caudal
cephalic
cyanosis
cytology
dermatologist
distal
epithelium
etiology
histology
lateral
leukemia
medial
megalomania
mucosa
pelvic
physiology
pleuritis
posterior
proximal
serosa
thoracotomy
ventral

SUFFIXES

pleurocentesis
erythrocyte
physiologist
ia (condition)
anemia
dermatitis
dermatology
gastromegaly
pelvimeter
pelvimetry
leukocytosis
acroparalysis
dermatopathy
cyanotic
mucous
anemic
duodenal
peritoneum
dermatology
cyanoderma
mucus

Information Frame ?? ?

1-1

The human body is a marvel in design. The shapes and textures of its structures are specifically designed for special functions. Ana/tom/y, from the Greek: ana (backward) + tome (cut) is the study of body structures. Physi/o/logy, from the Greek: physis (nature) + logos (study) is the study of body functions.

1-2

ana/tomy
a **nat'** o mē

Some early physicians studied human structures by dissecting dead bodies. This study of the body structures is called:

_____.

physi/o/logy
fiz ē **ol'** ō jē

Others studied how these structures worked or functioned. This science is called: _____.

1-3

word root
vowel
combining form
suffix

In the word physi/o/logy,
physi is the *_____;
o is the _____;
physi/o is the *_____;
and logy is the _____.

1-4

word root
vowel
combining form
suffix

Look up the word eti/o/logy in your dictionary. Eti/o/logy is the study of causes of disease. In this word:
eti is the *_____;
o is the _____;
eti/o is the *_____;
and logy is the _____.

ANSWER COLUMN

1-5

Good work! Now you are understanding the structure and function of medical language as well. Try these: -ist and -logist are suffixes for one who studies, a specialist. Use -ist as a suffix to build a word that means a person who studies the structures of the body:

ana/tom/ist
a **nat'** om ist

_____.

physi/o/logist
fiz ē **ol'** ō jist

Use -logist to build a word that means a person who studies the functions of the body: _____.

Information Frame ?

1-6

We often study the body using a structural organization, building from simple structures to more complex systems. Look at the table below to see the structural organization of the body.

STRUCTURE		DEFINITION
Cells		Unit structure of living things.
		Examples: leukocytes, erythrocytes, melanocytes
Tissues		Groups of cells organized for a common function.
		Examples: epithelial, connective, muscular, nervous
Organs		Groups of tissues organized for a common function.
		Examples: uterus, kidney, lungs, heart
Organ systems		Groups of organs organized for a common function.
		Examples: urinary, digestive, circulatory

ANSWER COLUMN

1-7

cell
sel

The smallest unit structure of living things is the _____.

1-8

word root
vowel
combining form

A word root like "cyt" plus a vowel like "o" makes the combining form **cyt/o.** In cyt/o, **cyt** is the *_____;
o is the _____; and **cyt/o** is the
*_____.

1-9

cyt/o

Use _____ as the combining form for cell.

1-10

cyt/o

More than 100 years ago, with the discovery of the microscope, scientists who studied tissues of plants and animals found that they were made of chambers they called cells. _____ is the combining form used to build words about cells.

1-11

cyt/o/logy
sī **tol'** ō jē

-logy is a suffix that means the study of. Build a word that means the study of cells. _____

ANSWER COLUMN

1-12

Cyt/o/logists study the cause of diseases of the cell, such as leukemia. The study of the cause of disease is

_____.

eti/o/logy
e tē **ol'** ə jē

1-13

-meter is a suffix meaning an instrument used to measure or count something. The instrument used to count cells is called a

_____. -metry is a suffix meaning the process of measuring or counting something. The process of counting cells is called _____.

cyt/o/meter
sīt **om'** et er
cyt/o/metry
sīt **om'** et rē

1-14

instrument

The word cyt/o/meter refers to the _____ used to measure or count. The word cyt/o/metry refers to the

process

_____ of measuring or counting.

1-15

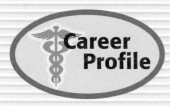

Career Profile

Cytotechnologists—prepare and screen human tissue slides to detect abnormalities. They are usually supervised by pathologists who are physicians that specialize in the study of disease.

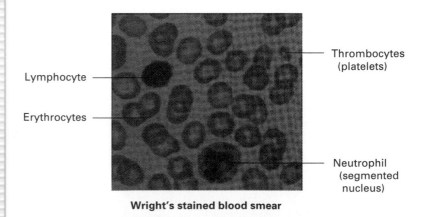

Lymphocyte

Erythrocytes

Thrombocytes (platelets)

Neutrophil (segmented nucleus)

Wright's stained blood smear

ANSWER COLUMN

	1-16
blast/o	A blast/o/cyte is an embryonic or immature cell. The combining form for embryonic or immature is _____. Think of this . . . when you have a "blast," you may act immature!
	1-17
blast	A cell in its embryonic or immature stage is called a _____.
	1-18
cell sel	-cyte may be used at the end of a word to indicate a type of cell. A leuk/o/cyte is a term referring to a type of white blood _____.
	1-19
immature or embryonic	-blast may be used at the end of a word to indicate an immature or embryonic cell. A hist/o/blast is a group of tissue cells that are * _____.
	1-20
hist/o/blast **his'** tō blast	Hist/o means tissues. Build a word that means: immature tissue _____; the study of tissues
hist/o/logy his **tol'** ə jē	_____; one who studies tissues
hist/o/logist his **tol'** ə jist	_____; a tissue cell
hist/o/cyte **his'** tō sīt	_____.

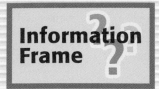

1-21

Membranes are thin sheets of tissue used to separate cavities, line cavities, cover organs, and line tubelike structures and vessels. Some membranes produce a fluid used to moisten the tissues to enable them to move easier and not stick to each other, or to help in the passage of substances through tubes and vessels.

Structure	Function	Location
Nerve	Control and communicate	Spinal nerves, cranial nerves, brain, neuroglia
Epithelium	Secrete and protect	linings of closed body cavities (serous), linings of open passageways (mucous), skin, and glands
Muscle (cardiac)	Move and protect	organs and vessels (smooth), heart (cardiac), skeleton (striated)
Connective tissue	Support and connect	bone, cartilage, tendons, ligaments, fascia, fat tissue

Four Types of Tissue and Their Functions

1-22

The **pleura** lines the pleural cavity around the lungs. The **peritoneum** lines the abdominal cavity. The **pericardium** lines the pericardial cavity around the heart. The pleura, peritoneum, and pericardium are all

membranes
mem' brānz

_____.

Locate these structures in the illustration showing the cavities and membranes on page 28. _____.

1-23

Now use what you have just learned.
The membrane surrounding the heart is the

peri/cardi/um
pair' ə **kar'** dē əm

_____.

The membrane surrounding the lungs is the

pleur/a
ploor' ə

_____.

The membrane lining the abdominal cavity is the

peri/toneum
pair' ə tŏ **nē'** əm

_____.

Good Job!

1-24

The linings of the closed body cavities are made of a type of epithelial membrane called a serous membrane or serosa. **ser/o** refers to serum, which is a body fluid similar to blood serum. Serous fluids are

ser/ous
ser' us

secreted by the _____ membranes.

1-25

The abdominal cavity is lined with a membrane called the

serous

peritoneum. The peritoneum is a _____ membrane.
The pleura is a membrane that surrounds the lungs. The pleura is a

serous

_____ membrane.

muc/ous

my$\overline{oo}$' cus

1-26

Mucous membranes, or mucosa, line open cavities and the structures of tubes, such as the nasal passages or intestinal tract, leading to the outside of the body. The intestinal mucosa is a type of
_____ membrane.

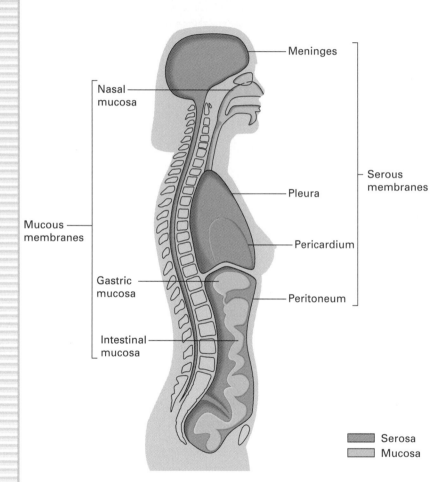

Mucous and serous membranes

ANSWER COLUMN

1-27

mucous

The respiratory tract is lined by the _____ membrane.

1-28

Skin is composed of epithelial-type tissue. **dermat/o** refers to the skin. When you see dermat or dermat/o, think immediately of

skin

_____.

1-29

A dermat/o/logist (dermatologist) is a specialist in a field of medi-

skin

cine. This person specializes in diseases of the _____.

1-30

In **dermat/o, dermat** is the

word root   *_____;

vowel   **o** is the _____;

combining form   and **dermat/o** is the *_____.

1-31

Dermat/itis means inflammation of the skin. The suffix that means

itis

inflammation is _____.

1-32

Signs of inflammation include redness, swelling, and heat. Dermatitis immediately forms a picture of red skin. To say that the skin is in-flamed, physicians use the word

dermat/itis

dûr mə **tī′**tis   _____.

1-33

Allergies are a common cause of red, swollen skin. This type of

dermat/itis

inflammation is called allergic _____.

ANSWER COLUMN

1-34

Acr/o/dermat/itis (acrodermatitis) is a word that means inflammation of the skin of the extremities. A person with red, inflamed hands has

acr/o/dermat/itis
ak rō dûr mə **tī'** tis

_____.

1-35

Acrodermatitis could result from stepping in a patch of poison ivy. A person with red, inflamed skin on his or her feet has

acrodermatitis

_____.

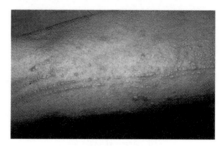

Contact dermatitis

1-36

Remembering the word acrodermatitis, which means inflammation of the skin of the extremities, draw a conclusion. -itis is a suffix that

inflammation

means _____.

1-37

acr/o is used to build words that refer to the extremities. To refer to extremities, physicians use words containing

acr/o or acr

*_____.

1-38

acr/o is found in words concerning the extremities, which in the human body, are the arms and legs. To build words about the arms,

acr/o

use _____.

NOTE: Think of an acrobat.

ANSWER COLUMN

1-39

The words acr/o/megaly (acromegaly), acr/o/cyan/osis (acrocyanosis), and acr/o/dermat/itis (acrodermatitis) all refer to the

extremities

_____.

1-40

megal/o means enlarged. Megal/o can also mean large. The suffix -megaly will mean something is

large, big, or   *_____.
   enlarged

1-41

Acr/o/megaly (acromegaly) means the extremities are

large, big, or   *_____.
   enlarged

1-42

Whenever organs become enlarged we may use the suffix -megaly or the combining form megal/o. Try this. Build two different words each meaning enlargement of the cardi/o heart

cardi/o/megaly   _____ or
kär′ de o **meg′** əl ē
megal/o/cardi/a   _____ /cardi/a
meg′ ə lo **kär′** de

1-43

word root   In **megal/o,** megal is the *_____;
vowel   **o** is the _____;
                   and **megal/o** is the
combining form   *_____.

1-44

The word that means a person has enlarged hands is

acr/o/megaly   _____.
ak rō **meg′** ə lē

1-45

-y is one suffix that makes a word a noun. Acromegaly is a

_____.

noun

1-46

cyan/o is used in words to mean blue or blueness. When photographers want to say something about how a film reproduces the color blue, they use *_____.

cyan/o or cyan

1-47

Dermat/osis means any skin condition. This word denotes an abnormal skin condition. The suffix that means condition is

_____.

osis

1-48

-osis: is a suffix
        forms a noun
        means disease or condition
Build a word that means a condition of blueness.

_____

cyan/osis
sī ə **nō′** sis

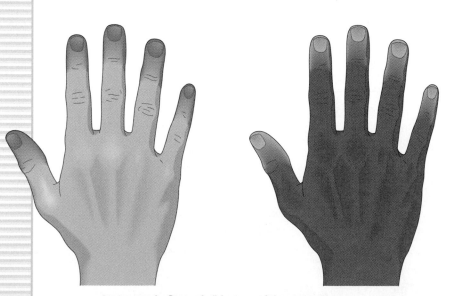

Acrocyanosis–Cyanosis (blueness of the extremities)

ANSWER COLUMN

---

cyan/o/tic
sī ə **nō′** tik

1-49

-tic is a suffix that forms an adjective. Build the term that means pertaining to a condition of blueness.

_____

---

cyan

1-50

Acr/o/cyan/osis means blueness of the extremities. The part of the word that tells you that the color blue is involved is

_____.

---

acr/o/cyan/osis
ak′ rō sī ə **nō′** sis

1-51

Acr/o/cyan/osis results from lack of oxygen. When the blood doesn't carry enough oxygen to the hands and feet,

_____ results.

---

osis

1-52

-osis is a suffix that makes a word a noun and means condition. To say a condition of blueness of the extremities, use the suffix

_____.

ANSWER COLUMN

1-53

paralysis in a word means loss of movement. Form a compound word meaning paralysis of the extremities.

acr/o/paralysis
ak′ rō pə **ral′** ə sis

_____

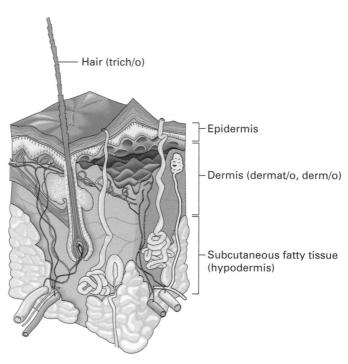

— Hair (trich/o)

Epidermis

Dermis (dermat/o, derm/o)

Subcutaneous fatty tissue (hypodermis)

Structures of the skin

1-54

Did you get it? If so, you are really learning medical terminology. (This one is for free.)

1-55

derm/o is another combining form for words referring to the skin; -pathy is a suffix meaning disease. Dermopathy means a disease condition of the _____.

skin

ANSWER COLUMN

blue skin or bluish dis-
coloration of the skin

noun

1-56

Derma is a word itself. It is a noun meaning skin. Cyan/o/derma is a
compound word. It means ** _____ and
is a _____ .
(noun/adjective)

1-57

thorac/ic
thor **a'** sik
pleur/al
plōō' əl
peri/card/ial
per i **kar'** dē əl
abdomin/al
ab **dom'** i nəl
pelv/ic
pel' vik

Study the diagram of the body cavities on page 37 and look for the
names and word roots of the cavities lined with serous type membranes. List the ventral cavities below:

chest: _____ cavity

lung: _____ cavity

heart: _____ cavity

abdomen: _____ cavity

pelvis: _____ cavity

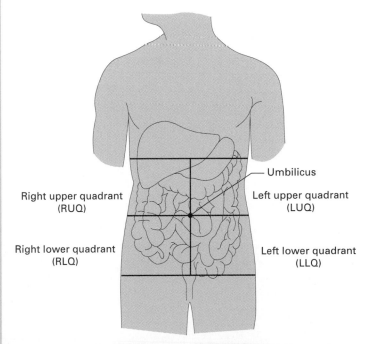

Umbilicus

Right upper quadrant
(RUQ)

Left upper quadrant
(LUQ)

Right lower quadrant
(RLQ)

Left lower quadrant
(LLQ)

Abdomen divided into quadrants

ANSWER COLUMN

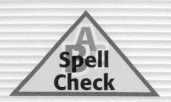

1-58

The word abdomen changes its spelling to **abdomin/o** for the combining form. Watch the switch from "e" to "i".

1-59

One method of identifying the location of symptoms of the abdomen, such as pain, is to divide the abdomen into quadrants. Study the illustration labeling the quadrants of the abdomen. Match the following abbreviations with the correct quadrant:

left lower quadrant

right lower quadrant

right upper quadrant

left upper quadrant

*LLQ _____ ;

*RLQ _____ ;

*RUQ _____ ;

*LUQ _____ ;

1-60

Thorac/o is the combining form for chest or thorax. -pathy is a suffix that comes from the Greek word "pathos" meaning disease or suffering. A general term for disease of the chest is

_____ .

thorac/o/pathy

thor' a **ko'** path ē

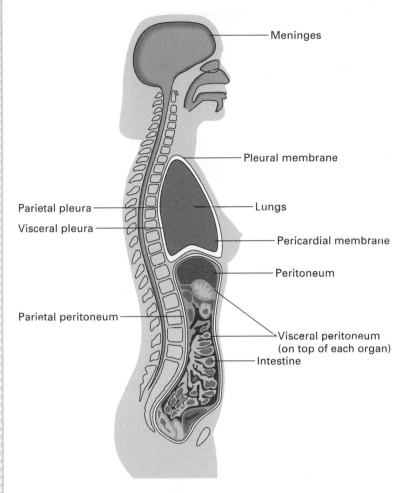

Meninges

Pleural membrane

Parietal pleura

Lungs

Visceral pleura

Pericardial membrane

Peritoneum

Parietal peritoneum

Visceral peritoneum
(on top of each organ)

Intestine

Dorsal and ventral cavity membranes

1-61

viscer/o is used to mean organ. The viscera (singular: viscus) are the internal organs of the body. Viscerad means toward the organs. Viscerogenic means growing organs. The combining form for organ is

_____.

viscer/o

ANSWER COLUMN

1-62

organs (internal)

In the words viscer/o/motor, viscer/o/pariet/al, and viscer/o/pleur/al, viscer/o refers to _____.

pariet/al
pa **rī'** e tal

Parietal means pertaining to the wall of an organ or cavity. The _____ pericardium is the membrane of the wall of the heart cavity.

1-63

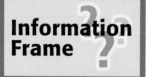
Information Frame

Uses of viscer/o and pariet/o:
visceral pleura   (membrane on the lung)
parietal pleura   (membrane on chest wall)
visceral peritoneum   (membrane on organs of the abdominal cavity)
parietal peritoneum   (membrane on abdominal cavity wall)
(PRONOUNCED: **vis'** er al; pa **rī'** e tal)

1-64

periton/eum
per' i tō **nē'** um

The membrane that lines the abdominal cavity is the _____.

periton/itis
per i tō **nī'** tis

Infection causing inflammation of the abdominal lining is _____.

1-65

Information Frame

The study of anatomy requires a common view of the body based on directions and locations and body position. We start with the body in what is called "anatomic position." Anatomic position is described as the person standing erect, facing forward, with the arms at their sides, and the palm side of the hands facing forward. The nose, belly, palms of the hands, and knees are all anterior. The occiput, wing blades (scapula), buttocks, and heels are all posterior.

ANSWER COLUMN

Try this.

1-66

Draw a figure standing in anatomic position and label the directions. You may use the illustration on page 41 to assist you.

1-67

Anatomical terms in English are taken from both Latin and Greek; therefore, you will see that many times there are two words for the same structure or direction. For example: anterior and ventral both mean front; posterior and dorsal both mean back.
Another word for anterior is

ventr/al
ven' trəl

_____.

dors/al
dor' səl

Another word for posterior is

_____.

1-68

Dors/al is one Greek term meaning back. Think of the large dorsal fin on a shark. The dorsal cavity includes the cranial and spinal cavities. When you want to indicate the back of the body you may use

dors/al
dor' səl

_____.

poster/ior
pōst **ēr'** ē ôr

Poster/ior is one Latin term meaning back. The back of the thigh is the _____ surface.

anter/ior
ant **ēr'** ē ôr

Ventr/al is a greek term for front. Can you deduce what the Latin term for front is? _____
Good!

Do it!

1-69

Study the table of directional terms below and their meanings. Then, locate each on the diagram showing directions of the body that follows this table.

Directional Word	Combining Form	Meaning
dorsal	dors/o	back, back side (posterior)
ventral	ventr/o	front, front side (anterior)
anterior	anter/o	front, front side (ventral)
posterior	poster/o	back, back side (dorsal)
cephalic	cephal/o	upward—toward the head
caudal, caudad	caud/o	downward—toward the tail (sacrum)
medial	medi/o	toward the midline
lateral	later/o	toward the side—away from the midline
superior	super/o	above (upper)
inferior	infer/o	below (lower)
proximal	proxim/o	near the point of origin or near the midline
distal	dist/o	away from the point of origin or away from the midline

ANSWER COLUMN

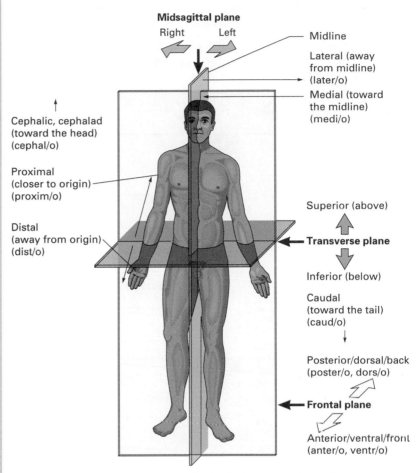

Midsagittal plane

Right   Left

Midline

Lateral (away
from midline)
(later/o)

Medial (toward
the midline)
(medi/o)

Cephalic, cephalad
(toward the head)
(cephal/o)

Proximal
(closer to origin)
(proxim/o)

Superior (above)

Distal
(away from origin)
(dist/o)

Transverse plane

Inferior (below)

Caudal
(toward the tail)
(caud/o)

Posterior/dorsal/back
(poster/o, dors/o)

Frontal plane

Anterior/ventral/front
(anter/o, ventr/o)

Directions and planes of the body in anatomic position.

1-70

Using the information about directional terms in the table, build
terms that mean pertaining to the:
front and side

anter/o/later/al
an' ter ō **lat'** er al

_____ ;

front and middle

anter/o/medi/al
 an' ter ō **mēd'** ē al

_____ ;

front and top

anter/o/super/ior
an' ter ō sup **ēr'** ē or

_____ .

ANSWER COLUMN

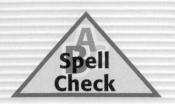

1-71

The combining forms for anterior and posterior do not include the "i." They are **anter/o** and **poster/o**.

1-72

back and side

poster/o/later/al
pōst' er ō **lat'** er al

_____;

back and outside

poster/o/extern/al
pōst' er ō eks **tern'** al

_____;

back and inside

poster/o/intern/al
pōst' er ō in **tern'** al

_____.

1-73

front and back (from front to back)

anter/o/poster/ior
an' ter ō pōst **ēr'** ē ôr,
or ventr/o/dorsal
vent' rō **dor'** sal

_____;

back and toward head

dors/o/cephal/ad
dor' sō **sef'** əl ad

_____;

toward the front

ventr/ad,
vent' rad,
or anter/ior
an **tēr'** ē ôr

_____;

middle and side

medi/o/lateral
mē' dē ō **lat'** er al

_____.

ANSWER COLUMN

1-74

Proximal means closer to a designated point (such as the origin of a muscle or limb), and **distal** means further from a designated point. Think of the words "approximate," meaning come close to estimating, and "distant," farther away from. Because the elbow is closer to the shoulder than to the hand, the elbow is

proxim/al
proks' i mal
dist/al
dis' tal

_____ to the hand. Because the ankle is further from the hip than the knee, the ankle is

_____ to the knee.

1-75

proximal

A fracture in the upper part of the femur (thigh bone) is a fracture of the _____ end of the femur.

1-76

distal

The bone in the tip of a finger (phalanx) is the _____ phalanx because it is farther from the origin of the finger.

1-77

middle and side
head to tail
back and above

After studying the table and diagram, you should be able to figure out the meanings of the following and write them below:
medi/o/lateral *_____
cephal/o/caudal *_____
poster/o/superior *_____
That's it. You have a great sense of direction.

The following medical abbreviations correspond to the terms in Unit 1.

Abbreviation	Meaning
A&P	anatomy and physiology
AP	anteroposterior
HCl	hydrochloric acid
LAT	lateral
LLQ	left lower quadrant
LUQ	left upper quadrant
PA	posteroanterior
RLQ	right lower quadrant
RUQ	right upper quadrant

You have been introduced to many new terms in this first unit. To make sure you know them well, work the review exercises on the following pages. Also, listen to the audio CD-ROM accompanying this third edition of *Medical Terminology Made Easy* and practice pronunciation.

**UNIT 1
REVIEW EXERCISES**

Review the terms you have learned in this unit by drawing the diagonal lines between the word parts and writing the meaning of each term. Use your medical dictionary or the frames if you need help. After you have completed these tasks, say each term aloud to practice pronunciation.

Part 1: Divide and Define

Example: 1. abdominopelvic   abdomin/o/pelv/ic—pertaining to the abdomen and pelvis

2. acrocyanosis   _____

3. acrodermatitis   _____

4. acromegaly   _____

5. acroparalysis   _____

6. anatomy   _____

7. anteroposterior   _____

8. cardiomegaly   _____

9. cephalocaudal   _____

10. cyanoderma   _____

11. cyanotic   _____

12. cytology   _____

13. cytometer   _____

14. cytometry   _____

15. dermatologist   _____

16. dermatopathy   _____

17. dermatosis   _____

18. distal   _____

19. dorsocephalad   _____

20. etiology   _____

21. gastromegaly   _____

22. mediolateral   _____

23. mucosa   _____

24. pericardium   _____

25. physiology   _____

26. pleura   _____

UNIT 1
REVIEW EXERCISES

27. proximal _____

28. serous _____

29. ventrodorsal _____

Part 2: Match each term with its correct meaning.

_____ 1. acromegaly   a. study of or pertaining to cause of disease

_____ 2. dermatology   b. adjective for blue condition

_____ 3. cyanoderma   c. lining of open cavities

_____ 4. dermatitis   d. the study of skin diseases

_____ 5. dermopathy   e. abnormally high platelet count

_____ 6. etiology   f. any disease of the skin

_____ 7. cytometry   g. study of body functions

_____ 8. acroparalysis h. enlarged extremities

_____ 9. anatomy   i. blueness of the skin

_____ 10. cyanotic   j. study of body structures

                         k. skin specialist

                         l. process of measuring cells

                         m. inflammation of the skin

                         n. paralysis of the extremities

Part 3: Write the medical term that means:

1. inflammation of the skin on the extremities_____

2. synonym for dorsal _____

3. below _____

4. to the side _____

5. pertaining to the chest _____

6. closer to the point of origin _____

7. pertaining to the lung cavity_____

8. general term for any skin disease _____

9. enlargement of the hands or feet _____

10. one who studies skin diseases_____

UNIT 1
REVIEW EXERCISES

Part 4: Use the medical terms listed below to complete these sentences:

acrocyanosis	paralysis	pericardium
cells	cytology	etiology
anterior	pelvic	lateral
inferior	dermatitis	histologist
distal	serous	mucosa

1. Tissues are groups of _____ organized for a common purpose.

2. The _____ department stains slides of cells for examination. Then, the _____ looks at the tissue to determine if the cell structure appears normal.

3. The _____ of the swimmer's _____ was a parasitic larva from bird droppings.

4. Because the fracture was located in the lower portion of the femur, it was described as a "complete fracture of the _____ portion of the femur."

5. The gastric _____ was irritated and bleeding as a result of the ulcer.

6. The pleural sac covering the lungs is a _____ type membrane.

7. The membrane that surrounds the heart is called the _____.

8. The _____ cavity is _____ to the abdominal cavity.

9. The _____ pituitary, located toward the front, produces many hormones that affect other glands.

10. The _____ malleolus is the portion of bone located on the outer side of the ankle.

UNIT 1
REVIEW EXERCISES

Part 5: Draw a line to match the abbreviation with its meaning.

1. A&P   anteroposterior

2. HCK   right upper quadrant

3. LLQ   posteroanterior

4. RUQ   left lower quadrant

5. AP   right lower quadrant

6. PA   hydrochloric acid

7. RLQ   left upper quadrant

                              hydrogen peroxide

                              anatomy and physiology

Part 6: From what you have learned about directional terms, complete the diagram below by labeling the blanks with the proper direction term or word part.

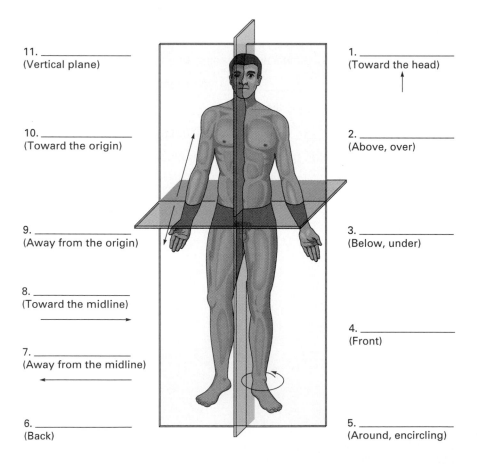

11. _____
(Vertical plane)

10. _____
(Toward the origin)

9. _____
(Away from the origin)

8. _____
(Toward the midline)

7. _____
(Away from the midline)

6. _____
(Back)

1. _____
(Toward the head)

2. _____
(Above, over)

3. _____
(Below, under)

4. _____
(Front)

5. _____
(Around, encircling)

Unit 1 Puzzle

As a self-test work the crossword puzzle and then check your answers in Appendix F.

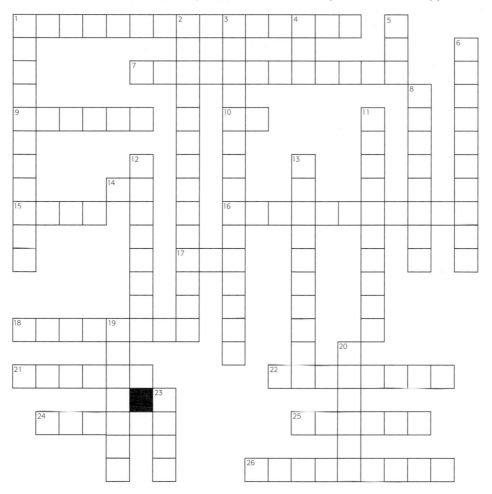

ACROSS

1. from back to front
7. from middle to side
9. tail end of the spine
10. anterior to posterior (abbrev.)
14. suffix for one who
15. suffix for inflammation
16. acro is the combining form
17. lateral (abbrev.)
18. pertaining to the head
21. chest
22. study of cells
24. type of membrane that secretes mucus
25. opposite of proximal
26. loss of movement

DOWN

1. membrane around the heart
2. pertaining to the abdomen and pelvis
3. surgical puncture of the chest
4. suffix for specialist
5. hydrochloride (chemical symbol)
6. destruction of tissue
8. front
11. the study of body functions
12. close to the origin
13. enlarged extremities
19. the study of body structures
20. back
23. suffix meaning condition

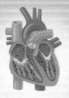

UNIT 2
Blood Cells, Cardiovascular, and Lymphatic Systems

Study these word parts, meanings, and examples. Then proceed to the first frame.

COMBINING FORMS

aneurysm/o (widening)
angi/o (vessel)
aort/o (aorta)
arteri/o (artery)
ather/o (thick fatty)
cardi/o (heart)
cyt/o (cell)
derm/o (skin)
dermat/o (skin)
ech/o (reflected sound)
electr/o (electricity)
erythr/o (red)
fibr/o (fibrous)
hem/o (blood)
hemat/o (blood)
isch/o (stopped flow)
leuk/o (white)
lip/o (fat)
lymph/o (lymph)
megal/o (enlarged)
melan/o (black)
phleb/o (vein)
radi/o (x-ray)
scler/o (hard)
son/o (sound)
thromb/o (clot)
tom/o (slice)
vas/o (vessel)

PREFIXES

brady- (slow)
tachy- (fast)

SUFFIXES

-algia (pain)
-ectomy (excision)
-emia (blood condition)
-genic (to generate)
-gram (picture)
-graph (recording instrument)
-graphy (process of making a picture)
-ia (noun- condition)
-y (noun- condition
-itis (inflammation)
-logist (one who studies)
-lysis (destruction)
-megaly (enlarged)
-oma (tumor)
-osis (condition)
-penia (low number)
-phobia (fear)
-plasty (repair)
-stasis (control or stopping)
-scope (looking instrument)
-scopy (process of using a scope)

Word Examples

COMBINING FORMS

aneurysm
angioplasty
aortogram
arteriostasis
atherosclerosis
cardiac
cytometry
leukoderma
dermatology
echocardiogram
electrocardiography
erythrocyte
fibroma
hemostasis
hematology
ischemia
leukocytopenia
lipoid
lymphatic
megalogastria
melanocyte
phlebotomy
radiology
arteriosclerosis
sonography
thrombosis
tomography
vasectomy

PREFIXES

bradycardia
tachycardia

SUFFIXES

cardialgia
thrombectomy
anemia
thrombogenic
radiogram
sonograph
echocardiography
leukemia
cardiomegaly
dermatitis
cardiologist
hematolysis
acromegaly
lymphoma
fibrosis
leukopenia
hematophobia
angioplasty
hemostasis
arterioscope
angioscopy

ANSWER COLUMN

2-1

NOTE: Most of these combining forms are used as prefixes (i.e., leukocyte).
Use this information for building words involving color

(Frames 2–2 through 2–8)	
leuk/o	white
melan/o	black
erythr/o	red
cyan/o	blue

2-2

Cyan/o/derma means blue skin. Build a word meaning:
red skin (blushing)

_____;

white skin

_____;

black (discolored) skin

_____.

(You draw the diagonal lines.)

erythr/o/derma
e rith′ rō **der′** mə′

leuk/o/derma
loo′ kō′ **der′** mə′

melan/o/derma
mel′ an ō der′ mə

2-3

Cyte (cyt/o) means cell. A histocyte is a tissue cell. Build a word meaning:
black cell (dark)

_____

white (blood) cell

_____

red (blood) cell

_____

melan/o/cyte
mel′ an ō sīt

leuk/o/cyte
loo′ kō sīt

erythr/o/cyte
e **rith′** rō sīt

ANSWER COLUMN

2-4

-emia means condition in the blood. Cyan/emia is blue blood. (Not literally in people; lobsters have blue blood.) Build a word involving the following colors when referring to blood conditions:
red (polycythemia) _____.

erythr/emia
e rith **rē'** mē ə
er' ith **rē'** mē ə

(too many red cells—red blood)

2-5

red
white
black

Erythr/o means _____.
Leuk/o means _____.
Melan/o means _____.

2-6

Cyanoderma sometimes occurs when children swim too long in cold water. A person who has a bluish discoloration of the skin for any reason suffers from

cyan/o/derma
sī' ə nō **der'** mə

_____.

2-7

In the compound word leuk/o/derma, the part that means white is _____.

leuk or leuk/o

ANSWER COLUMN

2-8

Leuk/o/derma means

white skin,
abnormally white skin,
whiteness of the skin,
etc.

* _____.

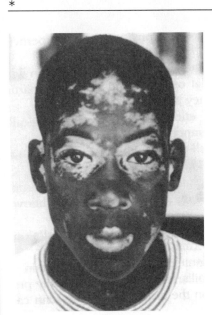

Vitiligo (leukoderma)

2-9

Recall that **cyt/o** refers to cells. A cell is the smallest structural unit of all living things. To refer to this smallest part of the

cyt/o

body, _____ is used.

2-10

Cytology is the study of cells. The part of cyt/o/logy that means

cyt/o

cells is _____.

2-11

Several kinds of cells are in blood. One kind is a leuk/o/cyte (refer to illustration on page 56). A measurement (counting) of cells is called cytometry. The instrument used to measure (count) cells is a

cells

cytometer. In each of these terms, **cyto** refers to _____.

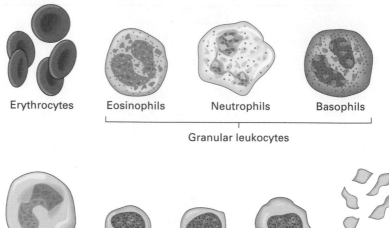

Erythrocytes   Eosinophils   Neutrophils   Basophils

Granular leukocytes

Monocytes   Small T   Small B   Plasma cell   Thrombocytes (Platelets)

Lymphocytes

Agranular leukocytes

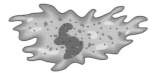

Wandering macrophage

Blood Cells and platelets

2-12

When physicians want to know the quantity of white blood cells per cubic millimeter (mm^3) of blood, they ask for a
_____ count (WBC).

leuk/o/cyte
lōo′ kō sīt

2-13

A differential white blood cell (Diff) count determines the percentage of different WBCs. Several kinds of leukocytes are in the blood. When physicians want to know how many of each type of leukocyte, they ask for a **differential** _____ count (Diff).

leuk/o/cyte

ANSWER COLUMN

2-14

Leuk/o/cyt/o/penia (leukocytopenia) means a decrease in the number of white blood cells. The part of the word that means **decrease in number** is _____.

-penia

2-15

"Penia" is the Greek word for poverty. The word that means **decrease in number** or **not enough** white blood cells is

_____.

leuk/o/cyt/o/penia
lōō′ kō sī tō **pē′** ne ə

2-16

You have heard of leuk/emia, popularly called "blood cancer." -em comes from a Greek word, "heme," meaning "blood." -ia is a suffix for condition. -emia is used to mean a blood condition. A noun meaning, literally, a condition of "white blood,"
is _____.

leuk/emia
lōō **kē′** mē ə

2-17

In leukemia, the blood is not really white. A laboratory finding of this disease is the presence of too many immature leukocytes in the blood. This finding was used to name the disease _____.

leukemia

2-18

If a blood vessel is blocked so that blood flow is stopped to tissues, this is called _____.

isch/emia
i **skē′** mē ə

2-19

-emia is a suffix that means *_____
_____.

condition of the blood
or in the blood

ANSWER COLUMN

2-20

Isch/emia (i **skē′** mē ə) is a condition in which blood flow is interrupted. Blood cancer (sign: abnormally increased leukocyte count) is called:

leuk/emia
lōō **kē′** mē ə

_____.

2-21

A transient isch/emic attack (TIA) is a temporary interruption

blood

of _____ flow.

2-22

Erythr/o means red. Erythr/emia literally means red blood, a synonym for polycythemia, in which there are too many red cells. Cells that contain a red substance (hemoglobin) are called red blood

erythr/o/cytes
e **rith′** rō sīts

cells, or _____.

2-23

A condition called polycythemia is also called

erythr/emia
e rith **rē′** mē ə

_____.

2-24

Abnormal bleeding can lead to a low red blood cell count. A patient who lacks the normal number of red blood cells suffers from

erythr/o/cyt/o/penia
e rith′ rō sīt ō **pē′** nē ə

_____.

2-25

Normal bleeding can lead to a low blood cell count.

-penia

Use the suffix _____ to indicate a low number.

ANSWER COLUMN

2-26

Blood clotting cells (thrombocytes) are also called platelets. A platelet count would be done to obtain the number of

thrombocytes

_____.

2-27

thromb/o means blood clot. The blood cells that

thromb/o/cytes
throm' bō sĭts
or platelets
plāt' lets

cause blood clots are _____.

2-28

Another type of blood cell is the **thromb/o/cyte**, also known as a platelet. Thrombocytes prevent bleeding by allowing the blood to clot. An abnormal decrease in the number of these clot-forming cells is

thromb/o/cyt/o/penia
thromb' ō sīt ō **pē'** nē ə

_____.

2-29

Look at the table indicating the test result values in a complete blood count (CBC) report. An abnormal increase in the number of white blood cells or leukocytes may be an indication of a bacterial infection. A low erythrocyte count indicates anemia. If there are not enough platelets, the blood may clot too slowly. The CBC is a valuable test because it tells us so much about the balance of blood cells related to overall health.

2-30

-osis may be used to indicate an increase in numbers of blood cells. Build a word that means an increase in

leuk/o/cyt/osis
lōō kō sī **tō'** sis
erythr/o/cyt/osis
e rith rō sī **tō'** sis
thromb/o/cyt/osis
thromb' ō sī **tō'** sis sī to'

white blood cells: _____;

red blood cells: _____;

platelets: _____.

COMPLETE BLOOD COUNT (CBC)
Specimen: Whole Blood

Test	Normal Average Values
Hgb (Hb)—Hemoglobin:	12–16 grams/100 milliliters
Hct—Hematocrit:	36–48% formed elements
RBC—Red Blood Cell Count:	4.2–6.2 million/mm^3
WBC—White Blood Cell Count:	5,000–10,000/mm^3
Platelet (Thrombocyte) Count:	350,000–450,000/mm^3

White Blood Cell Differential Count (Diff)—Wright's stain smear analysis based on 100 WBCs:

Neutrophil bands: 3–5%	Neutrophil Segs: 54–62%
Lymphocytes: 25–33%	Monocytes: 3–7%
Eosinophils: 1–3%	Basophils: 0–1%

Information Frame

2-31

The heart pumps blood through the body.

Think of these prefixes as you read about the layers of the heart and surrounding tissues:

Prefixes	Meanings
peri-	surrounding
epi-	upon
endo-	inside or inner

Recall that the peri/cardi/um is the membrane surrounding the heart and that the heart is located in the peri/cardi/al cavity. The epicardium is a membrane layer right on the heart, also called the visceral pericardium. Other layers of the heart include the muscle layer, or my/o/cardi/um, and the inner lining, or endo/cardi/um. See these labeled on the diagram of the heart on page 62.

ANSWER COLUMN

2-32

The muscle layer of the heart is the

my/o/cardi/um
mi o **kar'** de əm

_____.

The inner lining of the heart is the

endo/cardi/um
en do **kar'** de əm

_____.

The outer membrane right on the heart is the

epi/cardi/um
ep i **kar'** de əm

_____.

This may also be called the

peri/cardi/um
pair i **kar'** de əm

_____.

2-33

cardi/o (card/o) is used in building words that refer to the heart.
Card/itis means

inflammation of
   the heart

* _____

_____.

NOTE: When the suffix being used begins with a vowel, the
combining form is usually not required (i.e., card/itis, cardi/ectomy).
When the suffix being used begins with a consonant, a combining
form is usually required (i.e., cardi/o/dynia, cardi/o/logy).

2-34

Recall that -logy and -logist are suffixes:
logos—Greek for study
logy—noun, study of
logist—noun, one who studies
A cardi/o/logist is a specialist in the study of diseases of

heart

the _____.

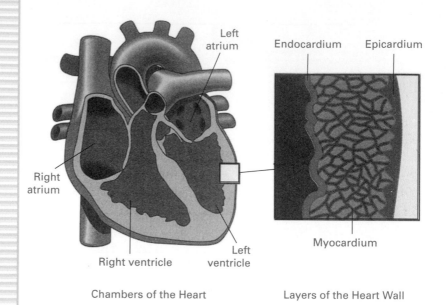

Chambers of the Heart   Layers of the Heart Wall

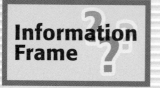

Information Frame

2-35

-ic and -ac are adjective suffixes. The following are adjectival forms of the words you have just learned:

leukem/ic
derm/ic
cyan/o/tic
leuk/o/cyt/ic
cardi/ac

2-36

A cardi/o/logist diagnoses heart diseases. The specialist who determines that a heart is diseased is a

_____.

cardi/o/logist
kär dē **ol′** ə **jist**

ANSWER COLUMN

2-37

A cardiologist may discover irregularities in the flow of the blood in the heart. The physician who performs cardiac catheterization

cardiologist

is a _____.

Use these suffixes for recording:

-gram   picture or record
-graph   instrument used to make a recording or picture
-graphy   process of using a recording instrument
-grapher   person who makes the recording or picture

2-38

-gram is the suffix meaning record or a picture. **electr/o** is the combining form for electrical. Give the meaning of

record of electrical
waves given off
by the heart (or
equivalent)

electr/o/cardi/o/gram. *_____

_____

_____

2-39

You will recall that -graph is a word root indicating an instrument used to make a recording or any pictorial device. An electr/o/cardi/o/gram is the record produced. An electrocardiograph is the instrument used to record the picture,

electr/o/cardi/o/gram
e lek′ trō **kär′** dē ō gram

or _____.

2-40

-graphy is a suffix for the **process** of making a recording (EKG or ECG). The electr/o/cardi/o/gram is a record obtained by the process of electr/o/cardi/o/graphy. A technologist can learn electrocardiography, but a cardiologist must read

electrocardiogram

the _____.

NOTE: The suffix -gram refers to the actual paper "read out" or picture on a computer screen. Think of obtaining a telegram from a telegraph.

ANSWER COLUMN

2-41

A physician can look at a graphic chart like this and learn something about a person's heart. The physician is a _____ and is reading an _____.

cardiologist
electrocardiogram

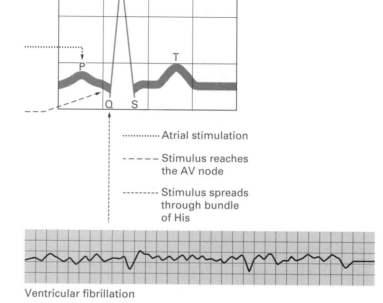

············ Atrial stimulation

– – – – Stimulus reaches the AV node

-------- Stimulus spreads through bundle of His

Ventricular fibrillation

Complete heart block (atrial rate, 107; ventricular rate, 43)

2-42

son/o is a combining form taken from the Latin word "sonus," meaning sound. A son/o/gram is a picture made by a sonograph. The process of obtaining the sonogram is called _____.

son/o/graphy
son **og'** ra fē
or
ultra/son/o/graphy
əl tra son **og'** raf ē

Note: The sonograph uses ultrasound which is sound waves beyond audible frequency to make images of the body.

ANSWER COLUMN

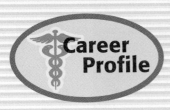

2-43

Registered diagnostic medical sonographers (RDMS) use ultra-sound (high-frequency waves) to create body images that are displayed on computerized monitors or to create still pictures showing shape and composition of organs and tissues.

2-44

The suffix -er means "one who." The person who performs sonography is called a _____.

son/o/graph/er
son **og'** ra fer

2-45

ech/o is a combining form meaning sound made by "reflected" sound waves. A **record** of sound waves reflected through the heart is an _____.

ech/o/cardi/o/gram
ek ō **kär'** dē ō gram

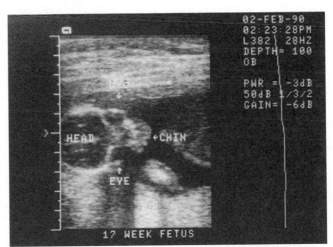

Fetal ultrasound (Prepared by Lynne Schreiber, BS, RDMS, RT[R])

ANSWER COLUMN

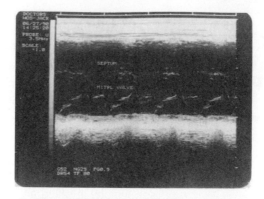

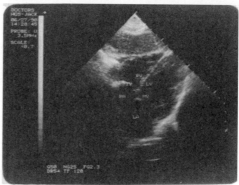

Echocardiogram (Prepared by Lynne Schreiber, BS, RDMS, RT[R])

2-46

The **process** of making the echocardiogram is called

_____.

ech/o/cardi/o/graphy
ek ō kär′ dē **og′** ra fē

2-47

radi/o is a combining form used to refer to radiation such as that used in x-rays. A picture made by using x-rays is called a _____.

radi/o/gram
rād′ ē ō gram

NOTE: Common use: an x-ray film is called a radiograph.

ANSWER COLUMN

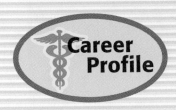

Career Profile

2-48

Radiation therapy technologists (RT[T]) use ionizing radiation applied to the body for treatment of disease. **Radiologic technologists (RT[R])** use x-rays to create images for diagnostic interpretation by physicians. Both professions position patients for exposure, operate x-ray equipment, and maintain records.

2-49

Build words for the following meanings: one who takes x-rays

radi/o/grapher
rād ē **og'** ra fer

_____.

one who studies (a physician specializing in) x-rays

radi/o/logist
rād ē **o'** lo jist

_____.

2-50

tom/o refers to slices or planes. An x-ray that takes views of slices or planes through the body is a tom/o/graph. The process is called

tom/o/graphy
tŏ **mog'** ra fē
tom/o/graphy

_____. A CT scan is

computed _____.

2-51

-algia is one suffix that means pain. Form a word that means heart pain. (Since -algia is a suffix, you will use the word root rather than the combining form.)

cardi/algia
kär dē **al'** jē ə

_____

2-52

Gastr/algia means pain in the stomach. When a patient complains of pain in the heart, this symptom is known
medically as _____.

cardialgia

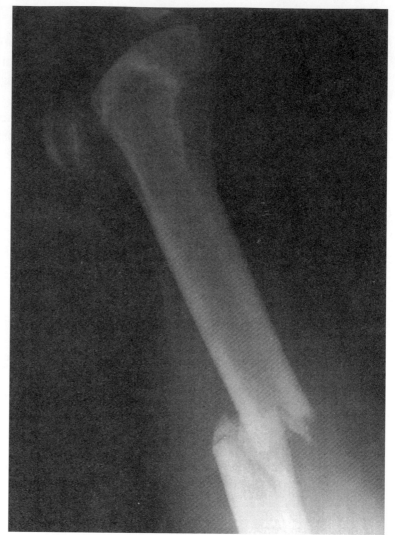

Radiograph: fractured femur (Prepared by Edwin Martin, BS, RT[R])

2-53

brady- is used in words to mean slow. Brady/cardia
means _____ heart action.

slow

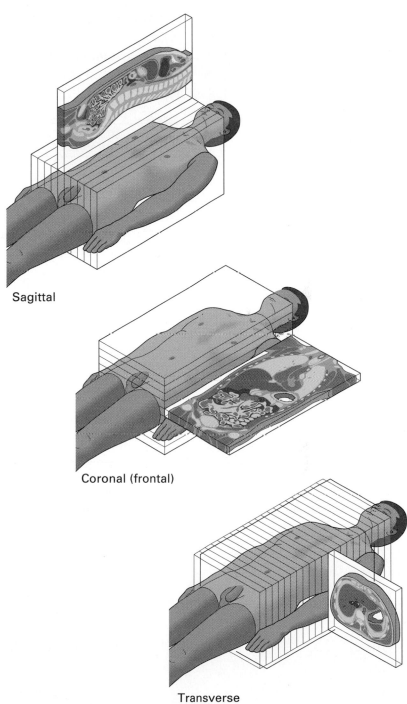

Sagittal

Coronal (frontal)

Transverse

Computed tomography (CT) planes

ANSWER COLUMN

Use the following table to experiment by mixing and matching word parts. Make up combinations and then look them up in your dictionary to see if they are real medical terms and what they mean. This information will also help you as you work frames 2–58 through 2–98.

Combining Forms	Suffixes
aort/o (aorta)	-gram (record, picture)
ather/o (thick like porridge, fatty)	-graph (instrument used to make a picture)
thromb/o (clot)	-graphy (process of recording a picture)
phleb/o (vein)	-plasty (surgical repair)
angi/o (vessel)	-blast (immature cell)
arteri/o (artery)	-osis (condition)
lymph/o (lymph)	-oma (tumor, growth)
aneurysm/o (aneurysm, widening)	-lysis (destruction, breakdown)
hem/o (blood)	-pathy (disease)
hemat/o (blood)	-stasis (control, stopping)
scler/o (hard)	-genesis, -genic (development, production)
fibr/o (fibrous)	-scope (instrument used to look)
	-scopy (process of using a scope)

ANSWER COLUMN

2-54

Arrhythmia is an abnormality of the heart beat. Abnormally slow heart action (below 60 bpm) is

brady/cardia
brad i **kär′** dē ə

_____.

Note: **bpm** is beats per minute.

2-55

tachy- is used in words to show the opposite of slow.
tachy- means *_____.

fast or rapid

2-56

Another type of arrhythmia is tachy/cardia.
Tachycardia means *_____.

rapid heart action

2-57

An abnormally fast heartbeat (above 100 bpm)
is called _____.

tachy/cardia
tak i **kär′** dē ə

2-58

Build a word meaning:
a generalized disease condition of the
vessels _____

angi/o/pathy
an jē **op′** ə thē

a generalized disease condition of lymph vessels

_____

lymph/angi/o/pathy
limf′ an jē **op′** ə thē

Surgical repair of a vessel

_____

angi/o/plasty
an′ jē ō plas′ tē

2-59

A (condition of) hardening is **scler/osis**. A hardening
of a vessel is _____.

angi/o/scler/osis
an′ jē ō sklə **rō′** sis

ANSWER COLUMN

2-60

It is possible to examine the inside of the blood vessels to detect blockages by looking with a instrument called an angi/o/scope. The process of performing this procedure is called angi/o/scopy. The suffix indicating the instrument used for the examination is

-scope

_____;

and the suffix indicating the procedure involving looking with this

-scopy

instrument is _____.

2-61

To look inside a vessel, a physician would use an

angi/o/scope
an' jē ō skōp

_____.

This procedure is called

angi/o/scopy
an jō **os'** kē pē

_____.

2-62

From what you have just learned, build a word that means:
an instrument used to look into an artery

arteri/o/scope
är **tir'** ē ō skōp

_____

the procedure of looking into an artery with a socpe

artri/o/scopy
är tir ē **os'** kō pē

_____.

Good job!

2-63

-oma is a suffix for tumor. A lymphatic tissue tumor

lymph/oma
limf **ō** mə

is _____.

A vessel tumor containing fibrous tissue is an

angi/o/fibr/oma
an jē o fī **brō'** mə

_____.

ANSWER COLUMN

2-64

The lymphatic system is a series of lymph vessels, lymph nodes, and organs that help circulate tissue fluids, absorb fats from the intestine, and fight infections by maturing cells called lymphocytes and producing antibodies.

When you see lymph/o think of the

lymphatic
lim **fa'** tik
_____ system.

2-65

Cells produced by the lymphatic system are called

lymph/o/cytes
lim' fō sītz
_____.

2-66

-lysis is a suffix meaning destruction. The destruction or breaking
angi/o/lysis
an jē **ol'** ə sis
down of vessels is _____.

2-67

Arteri/o is used in words about the arteries. Arteries are blood vessels that carry blood away from the heart. A word meaning hardening of the arteries is

arteri/o/scler/osis
är tir' ē ō sklə **rō'** sis
_____.

2-68

Arteri/o/scler/osis means hardening of the arteries. Build a word meaning:
a fibrous condition of the arteries

arteri/o/fibr/osis
är tir' ē ō fī **brō'** sis
_____

ANSWER COLUMN

2-69

ather/o means fatty or thick porridgelike or gruel. Hardening of the blood vessels (arteries) caused by a fatty substance (atheroma) is a condition called

ather/o/scler/osis
a′ ther ō skler **ō′** sis

_____.

2-70

-graphy is a suffix meaning the process of making a record (i.e., radiography). X-ray pictures are a type of record. For each term listed below, indicate the body part being x-rayed:

vessel   angi/o/graphy _____ ;
artery   arteri/o/graphy _____ .

2-71

Build a word meaning:
destruction (breakdown) of fat

lip/o/lysis   ____lip____o_____ ;
li **pol′**ə sis

destruction (breakdown) of cells

cyt/o/lysis   _____ .
sī **tol′**ə sis

2-72

hem/o refers to blood. A tumor of a blood vessel is a hem/angi/oma. (Note dropped **o**.)
An embryonic blood vessel cell is a

hem/angi/o/blast   _____ .
hem **an′** jē ō blast

A condition of blood in a joint is

hem/arthr/osis   _____arthr_____ .
hē mär **thrō′** sis, or
hēm är **thrō′** sis
hem/o/lysis   Destruction of blood is _____ .
hē mol′ ə sis

ANSWER COLUMN

2-73

hemat/o also refers to blood.
Another word for destruction of blood cells is

hemat/o/lysis
hē mə **tol'ə** sis

_____.

Phobia means fear.
An abnormal fear of blood is

hemat/o/phobia
hē mə tō **fō'** be ə

_____.

2-74

blood
hemat/o/logy
hē mə **tol'** ə je

Use hemat/o to mean _____.
The study of blood is _____.

One who specializes in the science of blood is a

hemat/o/log/ist
hē mə **tol'** ə jist

_____.

2-75

thromb/o is the combining form that means clot.
Thromb/o/angi/itis means inflammation of a vessel with

clot

formation of a _____.

2-76

-ectomy means to excise (surgically remove) or to cut out.

excision of a
  thrombus (clot)

Thromb/ectomy means ** _____.

2-77

The proper medical way to say clot is to say thrombus.

thrombus

A synonym for clot is _____.
NOTE: The plural of thrombus is thrombi.

ANSWER COLUMN

2-78

inflammation of
  a vein with clot
  formation

Thromb/o/phleb/itis means **_____

_____

_____.

2-79

Using thromb/o, build a word meaning:
a condition of forming a thrombus

thromb/osis
throm **bō′** sis

_____;

a cell that aids clotting

thromb/o/cyte
throm′ bō sīt

_____;

resembling a thrombus

thromb/oid
throm′ boid

_____ oid _____.

2-80

Deep vein thrombosis (DVT) is a condition that typically develops in
the large vessels of the leg. Vascular ultrasound may be performed
to detect a clot in a vein of the calf of the leg called deep vein

thromb/osis
throm **bō′** sis

_____.

2-81

Build a word meaning:
pertaining to the formation of a clot

thromb/o/gen/ic
throm bō **jen′** ik

_____ gen ____ ic _____;

destruction of a clot

thromb/o/lysis
throm **bol′** ə sis

_____;

lack of cells that aid in clotting

thromb/o/cyt/o/penia
throm bō sī tō **pē′** nē ə

_____.

ANSWER COLUMN

2-82

A thrombus may block, or "occlude," a vessel. This occlusion may cause ischemia, stopping blood supply to the tissues, producing an infarct (necrosis of tissue). If this happens in the heart muscle, the condition is called myocardial infarction (MI). When blood flow is stopped to an area of tissue, this is called _____.

isch/emia
i **skē'** mē ə

2-83

Look it up!

Look up the following terms in your medical dictionary and write their definitions below:

occlusion *_____
_____;
infarct *_____
_____;
myocardial *_____
_____.

2-84

A thrombus or piece of a thrombus may move through blood vessels to another part of the body. This moving thrombus is called an **embolus** or embolism. An embolus may cause a block in a vessel called an _____.
Lack of blood flow to an area is called
_____. A moving blood
clot is called an _____.

occlusion
ō **kloo'** shun
isch/emia
embolus
e**m'** bō ləs
or
embolism
e**m'** bō lizm

ANSWER COLUMN

my/o/cardi/al
    in/farct/ion
mī ō **kär′** dē əl
in **fark′** shun

2-85

If an artery of the heart muscle is occluded and an area
of tissue has no blood supply, a *_____.
_____ may occur.

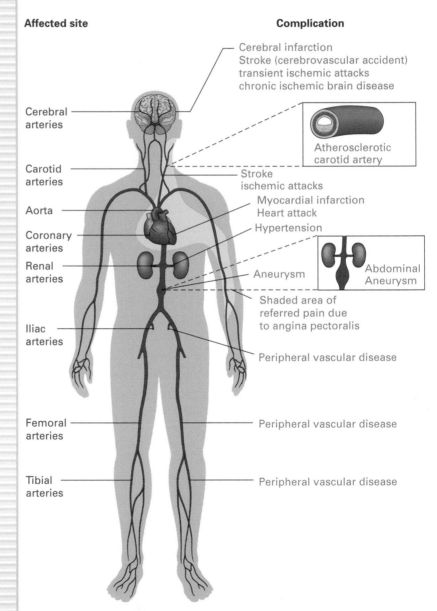

Affected site

Cerebral
arteries

Carotid
arteries

Aorta

Coronary
arteries

Renal
arteries

Iliac
arteries

Femoral
arteries

Tibial
arteries

Complication

Cerebral infarction
Stroke (cerebrovascular accident)
transient ischemic attacks
chronic ischemic brain disease

Atherosclerotic
carotid artery

Stroke
ischemic attacks

Myocardial infarction
Heart attack

Hypertension

Abdominal
Aneurysm

Aneurysm

Shaded area of
referred pain due
to angina pectoralis

Peripheral vascular disease

Peripheral vascular disease

Peripheral vascular disease

Arteries affected by atherosclerosis and resulting complications

ANSWER COLUMN

2-87

"Vas" is a Latin word root meaning vessel. The term for pertaining to vessels, especially blood vessels, is "vascular." The vascular

vessels

system refers to blood _____.

2-88

Arteries and veins are part of a system of vessels that carry blood called

vascular
vas′ kyōō lər

the _____ system. Use the combining form **cardi/o** for heart and vascular to build a term pertaining to the blood vessels supplying the heart:

cardi/o/vascular
kär dē ō **vas′** kyōō lər

_____.

2-89

A registered vascular technologist (RVT) uses sonography to examine blood vessels for abnormalities. One condition a RVT might find is a widening caused by a weakening in an artery wall, called an aneurysm. A widening of the abdominal

aneurysm
an′ yoor izm

aorta would be an aortic _____.

2-90

Continued weakening of the blood vessel wall because of aneurysm may lead to rupture of the vessel. A cardiovascular aneurysm that ruptures may be the cause of a heart attack. Hypertension (high blood pressure) and atherosclerosis are conditions that may lead to vessel

aneurysm

weakening, or _____, and then heart attack.

2-91

The term "aneurysm" is a tricky one to spell and say.
The "eu" is a diphthong, with the "e" silent and the "u" pronounced.
Then, instead of an "i," a "y" is used. Practice writing "aneurysm":

Spell Check

_____.

ANSWER COLUMN

2-92

Arteries (arteri/o) are vessels (angi/o) that carry blood away from the heart. Veins are vessels that carry blood

heart

back to the _____.

2-93

A combining form for vein is **phleb/o**. Arteriosclerosis is

arteries

hardening of the _____. Hardening

phleb/o/scler/osis

of veins is called _____.

fleb′ ō sklə **rō′** sis

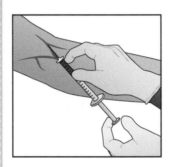

Venipuncture

2-94

Build a word meaning:
excision of a vein

phleb/ectomy

_____ ectomy _____;

fli **bek′** tə mē

incision into a vein (venipuncture)

phleb/o/tomy

_____ tomy _____;

fleb **ot′** ə mē

inflammation of a vein

phleb/itis

_____ itis _____.

fleb **ī′** tis

ANSWER COLUMN

2-95

-plasty is a suffix meaning repair. Think of
a plastic surgeon. Phleb/o/plasty means

surgical repair of
  a vein

*_____.

Phleb/o/tomy means

incision into a vein
  or venipuncture

*_____.

2-96

-Stasis means the act or condition of stopping or controlling.
Hem/o/stasis means

act of controlling
  blood flow

*_____

phleb/o/stasis
fli **bos'** tə sis

_____. A word meaning: control
of flow in veins is _____;

arteri/o/stasis
är tir' ē **os'** tə sis

control of flow in arteries is

_____.

2-97

Complete each phrase below:

blood

hemostasis means control in the flow of _____;
phlebostasis means control in the flow through

veins

_____;
arteriostasis means control in the flow through

arteries

_____.

2-98

Build a word meaning:

lymph/o/stasis
lim **fos'** tə sis

control of lymph flow _____.

NOTE: Although the formal pronunciation of words using -stasis is
shown above, a more common pronunciation is also acceptable, i.e.,
hemostasis (hē mō **stā'** sis), lymphostasis (lim fō **stā'** sis).

ANSWER COLUMN

The following medical abbreviations correspond to the terms in Unit 2.

Abbreviation	Meaning
AA	aortic aneurysm
AMI	acute myocardial infarction
AS	arteriosclerosis
ASCVD	arteriosclerotic cardiovascular disease
ASHD	arteriosclerotic heart disease
BPM	beats per minute
CABG	coronary artery bypass graft
CAT, CT	computed (axial) tomography
CBC	complete blood count
CHF	congestive heart failure
Diff	differential white blood cell count
DVT	deep vein thrombosis
ECHO	echocardiogram
ECG, EKG	electrocardiogram
HcT	hematocrit
HGB, HB, Hgb, Hb	hemoglobin
MI	myocardial infarction
P	pulse
PAT	paroxysmal atrial tachycardia
PVC	premature ventricular contraction
RBC	red blood cell (count)
RDMS	Registered Diagnostic Medical Sonographer
RT(R)	Radiographic Technologist (Registered)
RT(T)	Registered Radiologic Technologist (Therapist)
RVT	Registered Vascular Technologist
TIA	transient ischemic attack
VFib (VF)	ventricular fibrillation
WBC	white blood cell (count)
XR	x-ray

You have been introduced to many new terms in this unit. To make sure you know them well, work the review exercises on the following pages. Also, listen to the CD-ROM accompanying the third edition of *Medical Terminology Made Easy* and practice pronunciation.

UNIT 2
REVIEW EXERCISE

Part 1: Review the terms you have learned in this unit by drawing the diagonal lines between the word parts and writing the meaning of each term. Use your medical dictionary or the frames if you need help. After you have completed these tasks, say each term aloud to practice pronunciation.

1. aneurysm _____

2. angiography _____

3. angiolysis _____

4. arteriosclerosis _____

5. bradycardia _____

6. cardialgia _____

7. cardiologist _____

8. cardiovascular _____

9. carditis _____

10. cytolysis _____

11. echocardiography _____

12. electrocardiogram _____

13. erythremia _____

14. erythroderma _____

15. hematophobia _____

16. hemolysis _____

17. hemostasis _____

18. ischemia _____

19. leukocytosis _____

20. lymphangiopathy _____

21. lymphoma _____

22. melanocyte _____

23. myocardial _____

24. phlebosclerosis _____

25. phlebotomy _____

26. radiographer _____

27. sonography _____

UNIT 2
REVIEW EXERCISE

28. tachycardia   _____

29. thrombectomy   _____

30. thrombocytopenia   _____

31. thrombogenic   _____

Part 2: Match each term with its correct meaning.

_____ 1. bradycardia   a. pertaining to the heart muscle

_____ 2. myocardial   b. control of blood flow

_____ 3. thrombolysis   c. blood clotting cell

_____ 4. angiography   d. instrument used to picture electrical activity of the heart

_____ 5. phlebectomy   e. heart specialist

_____ 6. hemostasis   f. one who makes pictures of organs using sound waves

_____ 7. lymphangitis   g. inflammation of a gland

_____ 8. cardiologist   h. destruction of blood clots

_____ 9. sonographer   i. abnormally slow heart rate

_____10. electrocardiograph   j. inflammation of a lymph vessel

     k. abnormally slow breathing

     l. process of x-raying a vessel

     m. excision of a vein

     n. the study of pain and sensation control

Part 3: Write the medical term that means:

1. the process of using reflected sound to test heart function_____

2. pain in the heart _____

3. abnormally fast heart rate_____

4. hardening of the arteries _____

5. blood clot causing inflammation of a vein _____

6. pertaining to producing blood clots_____

7. tumor of lymph tissue _____

8. destruction of blood _____

9. blood vessel tumor _____

10. general term of any disease of the vessels _____

UNIT 2
REVIEW EXERCISE

Part 4: Use the medical terms listed below to complete these sentences:

tachycardia	leukocytopenia	melanocytes	cardiologist
ischemic	cytolysis	thrombus	radiographer
sonography	leukoderma	thrombocytes	leukocytosis

1. John applies make-up to even out his skin color because he has a disease that causes lack of pigment or white patches of skin called _____. The _____ are the pigment cells that are affected by this disease.

2. If the normal WBC count is 5,000–10,000/mm³ of blood and the patient has 2,500 indicated on the CBC report, this condition is called _____, and may indicate a viral infection. A bacterial infection would cause _____, indicated by a high WBC count.

3. Mrs. O'Conner has hypertension and is experiencing a temporary loss of blood to a part of the brain causing dizziness and blurred vision. The physician suspects a TIA, or transient _____ attack.

4. A chemical agent that destroys red blood cells is added to blood before counting the WBCs, causing _____.

5. A synonym for platelets is _____.

6. When an injury occurs, platelets cause a _____ to form to stop the bleeding.

7. The physician _____ reads and interprets the mounted EKG tracing.

8. Fetal _____ is performed to detect abnormalities before birth.

9. The radiologist instructs the _____ on proper positioning of the patient for obtaining good quality x-rays.

10. If a patient has a resting heart rate of 130 bpm, compared to normal of 72 bpm, he or she is experiencing _____.

UNIT 2
REVIEW EXERCISE

Part 5: Match the abbreviation on the left with its correct meaning on the right by drawing a line.

1. CABG   acute myocardial infarction

2. Diff   hematocrit

3. HGB   premature ventricular contraction

4. AMI   aortic aneurism

5. TIA   WBC differential

6. XR   complete blood count

7. CBC   hemoglobin

8. HCT   coronary artery bypass graft

9. AA   transient ischemic attack

10. PVC   radiogram

UNIT 2
REVIEW EXERCISE

Part 6: Label the arteries indicated in this diagram. Then draw a line to the corresponding circulatory system disorder listed.

peripheral vascular disease
aneurysm
stroke
transient ischemic attack
angina
hypertension
myocardial infarction

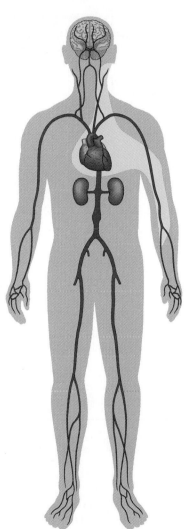

Unit 2 Puzzle

As a self-test work this crossword puzzle and then check your answers in Appendix F.

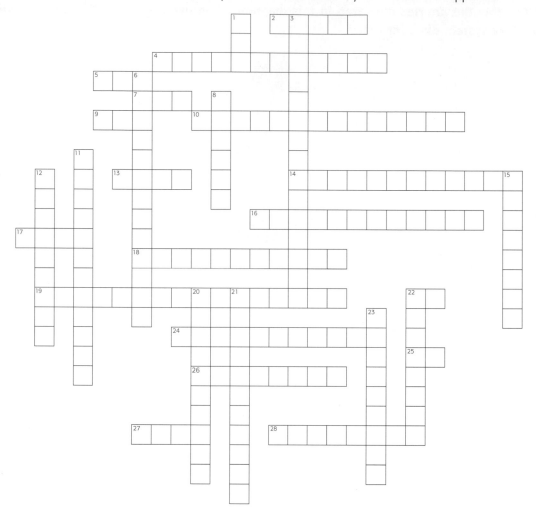

ACROSS

2. prefix meaning fast
4. fear of blood
5. transient ischemic attack (abbrev.)
7. radiographic technologist (registered)
9. registered vascular technologist
10. blood vessels and heart
13. WBC differential
14. lymph vessel tumor
16. destruction of blood clots
17. combining form—slices
18. surgical repair of a vessel
19. hardening of the arteries
22. myocardial infarction (abbrev.)
24. slow heart rate
25. aortic aneurysm
26. lack of blood flow to an area
27. coronary artery bypass graft
28. lymphatic tumor

DOWN

1. hematocrit
3. fatty deposits in vessels
6. control of artery flow
8. combining form for heart
11. too many WBCs
12. ultrasound instrument
15. widening of a vessel
20. heart ache
21. inner lining of the heart
22. melanocyte tumor
23. study of diagnostic images (x-ray)

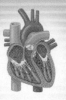 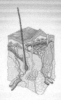

UNIT 3
Nervous System and Tumors

Study these word parts, meanings, and examples. Then proceed to the first frame.

COMBINING FORMS
aden/o (gland)
ather/o (fatty, porridge-like)
carcin/o (cancer)
cephal/o (head)
cerebr/o (cerebrum)
emes/is (vomiting)
encephal/o (brain, inside the head)
epitheli/o (epithelial)
fibr/o (fibrous)
hist/o (tissue)
lei/o (smooth)
lip/o (fat)
lymph/o (lymphatic)
melan/o (dark pigmented)
mening/o (meninges)
my/o (muscle)
myel/o (spinal cord)
nat/o (birth)
ne/o (new)
neur/o (nerve)
onc/o (tumor)
oste/o (bone)
papill/o (small elevation of tissue)
pariet/o (wall)
periton/o (peritoneum)
pleur/o (lung)

psych/o (mind)
rhabd/o (rod shaped)
spin/o (spinal)
viscer/o (organ)

PREFIXES
anti- (against)
dys- (difficult, painful)
hydro- (water)
neo- (new)

SUFFIXES
-algia (noun), algic (adjective), pain
-blast (embryonic or immature)
-cele (hernia)
-ectomy (excision)
-genesis (generate, develop)
-malacia (softening)
-oid (like, resembling)
-oma (tumor, abnormal growth)
-ous (adjective) (material, condition)
-pathy (disease)
-plasia (development)
-plasm (growth of tissue)
-tomy (incision)
-trophy (development)
-tropic (affecting)

Word Examples

COMBINING FORMS

adenopathy
atherosclerosis
carcinoma
cephalalgia
cerebrospinal
hyperemesis
encephalocele
epithelial
fibroid
histology
leiomyoma
lipoma
lymphatic
melanocyte
meningitis
myospasm
prenatal
neoplasm
neurosurgeon
oncologist
osteopathy
papilloma
parietal
peritoneum
pleura
psychology

rhabdomyosarcoma
spinal
visceral

PREFIXES

antineoplastic
dysplasia
hydrocephalus
neonatal

SUFFIXES

neuralgia
myoblast
meningocele
atherectomy
oncogenic
osteomalacia
mucoid
carcinoma
serous
hypoplasia
ecephalopathy
neoplasm
cerebrotomy
dystrophy
psychotropic

ANSWER COLUMN

3-1

Neur/o refers to nerves. Neur/o/logy, the study of the nervous system, includes the study of the anatomy and physiology of the brain, spinal cord, and nerves. A neur/o/logist is a physician specialist who treats diseases of the nervous system. The study of the nervous system is called _____.

neur/o/logy
noor **ol′** ō jē

3-2

A specially trained physician performs surgery on the structures of the nervous system. This specialist is called a

_____.

neur/o/surgeon
noor ō ser′ jən

3-3

Use the suffixes you have already learned to build words that mean:
inflammation of a nerve

neur/itis
noor **i′** tis

_____;

destruction of nerve tissue

neur/o/lysis
noor **ol′** ə sis

_____;

any disease involving nerves

neur/o/pathy
noor **op′** ə thē

_____.

Good work!

3-4

In Greek mythology, Psyche was the beautiful daughter of a mortal king, with whom Cupid, a god, fell in love. She was the personification of fervent emotion, and her story represents the triumph of the spirit or soul. The combining form psych/o is used in words that refer to the functions of the mind and mental processes as compared to the physical nervous system. Psych/o/logy is the study of the

mind or mental processes

* _____.

ANSWER COLUMN

3-5

A psych/o/logist is a person who studies

psych/o/logy
sī **kol'** ō jē
_____.

3-6

Psych/o/therapy is the process of treating mental disorders using words, art, drama, or movement to express feelings. A clinical psych/o/logist helps clients by treating them using

psych/o/therapy
sī kō **ther'** ə pē
_____.

3-7

Psych/o/therapy is also used by psych/iatrists. A psych/iatrist is a physician (MD or DO) who specializes in treatment of patients with mental illness. Patients who need medication and admission to a hospital would be treated by a

psych/iatrist
sī **kī'** ə trist
_____.

3-8

Use what you have learned to build a word that means: physician that treats mental illness

psych/iatrist
_____;

psych/o/logy
the study of mental processes

_____;

3-9

At this stage of word building, students sometimes find that they have one big pain in the head. The word for pain in the head, commonly called a headache, is cephal/algia. The word root for head is

cephal
_____.

ANSWER COLUMN

---

algia

3-10

One suffix for pain is _____.

---

cephal/algia
sef ə **lal'** jē ə

3-11

If you are suffering from cephalalgia, persevere, for later this gets to be fun. Any pain in the head may be called

_____.

---

adjective

ic

3-12

Cephal/ic means pertaining to or toward the head.
Cephal/ic is a(n) _____ (noun/ adjective). This is evident because cephalic ends in

_____.

---

cephalic

3-13

In the phrase "lack of cephalic orientation," the adjective is _____.

---

water or fluid
or
watery fluid

3-14

A hydr/o/cyst is a sac (or bladder) filled with watery fluid. Hydr/o is used in words to mean
* _____.

---

hydr/o/cephalus
hī drō **sef'** ə lus

3-15

Hydr/o/cephalus is characterized by an increased amount of fluid (cerebrospinal fluid) in the skull. A collection of fluid in the head is called _____.

ANSWER COLUMN

3-16

Hydrocephalus, unless treated by surgery, results in deformity. The face seems small, eyes are abnormal, and the head enlarges.

Hydrocephalus

_____ may also cause brain damage.

3-17

Because of the damage to the brain that may result if untreated, children with _____

hydrocephalus

may develop mental impairment.

3-18

Hydrocephalus is the noun. The adjectival ending is -ic.

Hydr/o/cephal/ic

_____ children receive

hī drō sə **fal'** ik

special training in schools for the mentally impaired.

Dictionary exercise:
Look up the following terms in your Medical Dictionary and compare their meanings:
hydrocephalus _____
hydrocephaly _____
hydrencephalus _____

ANSWER COLUMN

encephal/itis
en sef′ ə lī′ tis

3-19

Inside the head, **en**closed in bone, is the brain; **encephal/o** is one term used in words pertaining to the brain. Build a word meaning inflammation of the brain.

_____

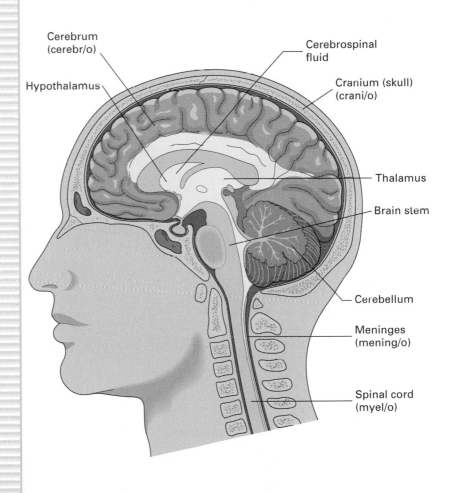

Cerebrum
(cerebr/o)

Cerebrospinal
fluid

Hypothalamus

Cranium (skull)
(crani/o)

Thalamus

Brain stem

Cerebellum

Meninges
(mening/o)

Spinal cord
(myel/o)

3-20

The suffix for tumor is -oma. Use what is necessary from encephal/o to build a word for brain tumor.

_____

ANSWER COLUMN

3-21

The Greek word for "hernia" is "kele"; the suffix is -cele.
Encephal/o/cele is a word meaning herniation of

brain

_____ tissue.

3-22

An encephalocele occurs when some brain tissue protrudes through
a cranial fissure. The word for herniation of brain tissue is

encephal/o/cele
en **sef'** ə lō sēl

_____.

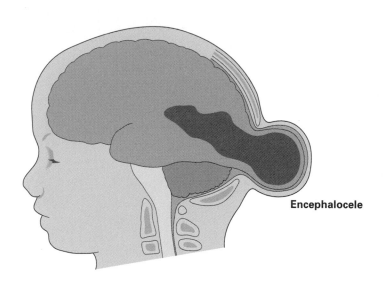

Encephalocele

3-23

Any hernia is a projection of a part from its natural cavity. Herniation
is indicated by -cele. A projection of brain tissue from its natural cavity is an

encephalocele

_____.

3-24

Malacia is a word meaning softening of a tissue.
Encephal/o/malacia means *_____

softening of
brain tissue

_____.

ANSWER COLUMN

3-25

malac/o is the combining form. The word root is

malac   _____.

3-26

Recall that -ia is a suffix that forms a noun, meaning condition. A
noun meaning softening of brain tissue is

encephal/o/malacia   _____.
en sef′ ə lō mə **lā′** shə

3-27

Some brain diseases can also cause softening and produce the condition called

encephalomalacia   _____.

3-28

-tomy is used as a suffix for making an incision (cutting into). An incision into the brain is an

encephal/o/tomy   _____.
en sef ə **lot′** ō mē

3-29

From your knowledge of the word parts **electr/o**, **encephal/o**, and
-gram, build a term meaning: picture of the electrical activity of the
brain

electr/o/encephal/o/gram   _____.
ē lek′ trō en **sef′** ə lō gram

3-30

The process of recording electrical brain activity is called

electr/o/encephal/o/graphy _____.
ē lek′ trō en sef′ ə **log′** ra fē

ANSWER COLUMN

3-31

You can form words without knowing the meaning in the next three frames. Use what is needed from encephal + itis to form
a word: _____.

encephal/itis

3-32

Use what is needed from   encephal/o
                            mening
                            -itis

encephal/o/mening/itis
en sef′ ə lō men in **jī′** tis

_____.

3-33

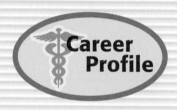
Career Profile

Electroneurodiagnostic (END) technologists are allied health professionals who perform electroencephalograms (EEG), evoked potentials (EP), polysomnograms, (PSG), nerve conduction studies (NCS), and electronystagmograms (ENG). The END technologist works under the supervision of a physician who is responsible for interpretation and clinical correlation of the results. Individuals entering the END profession may be a graduate of a Committee on Accreditation of Allied Health Education Program (CAAHEP)–accredited associate degree program and take a national certification examination in electroneurodiagnostic technology developed by the American Board of Registration of EEG and EP technologists.

3-34

The study of brain wave activity, whether awake or asleep, is the work of physicians assisted by the

electr/o/neur/o/diagnos/tic
ē lek′ trō nōō′ rō
dī əg **nos′** tik

_____.

(END) technologist.

3-35

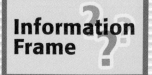
Information Frame

Look up myel/itis in your dictionary. From the definition, you conclude that **myel** is the word root for spinal cord and bone marrow.

ANSWER COLUMN

3-36

Use what is needed from   encephal/o
                          myel/o
                          -pathy

encephal/o/myel/o/pathy
en sef′ ə lo‾ mī əl **op′** ə thē

_____.

3-37

Find the word myeloblast in your dictionary. Write the

bone marrow or spinal cord   meaning below. *_____
germ cell
myel/o   _____

                                 The combining form of **myel** is _____.

3-38

Find a word meaning:
pertaining to myelocytes

myel/o/cyt/ic
mī′ el ō **sit′** ik   _____;

myel/o/cele   herniation of the spinal cord
mī′ el ō sēl
                                 _____.

3-39

Information Frame

Poliomyelitis is caused by a viral infection that inflames the tissues of
the spinal cord and brain and affects their ability to send nerve mes-
sages to the muscles. Respiratory as well as skeletal muscles are affected, endangering a person's life and causing paralysis. This disease
is prevented by vaccination with inactivated polio vaccine (IPV), administered by injection. Poliomyelitis still affects people in countries
where vaccination has not been available.

3-40

In the disease poli/o/myel/itis, the word part indicating that the

myel   spinal cord is affected is _____.

ANSWER COLUMN

3-41

-plas/ia means development or formation. This kind of formation occurs naturally instead of being done by a plastic surgeon. Hyper/plasia is an increase in the number of cells in a tissue (i.e., tumor). Dys/plas/ia means

defective (poor or
abnormal) formation

*_____

_____.

3-42

myel/o/dys/plasia
mī′ ə lō dis **plā′** zhə

Build a term that means defective (abnormal) formation of the spinal cord: _____.
(body part + disorder)

3-43

A/plasia means failure of an organ to develop properly. A word that means overgrowth or too much development is

hyper/plasia
hī per **plā′** zhə

_____.

3-44

Hypo- is the opposite of hyper-. If overdevelopment is hyperplasia, underdevelopment is expressed as

hypo/plasia
hī pō **plā′** zhə

_____.

3-45

A prefix goes in front of a word to change its meaning. In the words hyper/trophy, hyper/emia, and hyper/emesis, hyper- changes the meaning of trophy, emia, and emesis.

prefix

hyper- is a _____.

3-46

hyper- is a prefix that means above or more than normal. To say that a person is overly critical, you would

hyper

use the word _____critical.

ANSWER COLUMN

3-47

Emesis refers to vomiting. Excessive vomiting is called

hyper/emesis
hī per **em'** ə sis

_____.

| Normal size and number | Hyperplasia increased numbers | Hypertrophy increased size | Hypertrophy and hyperplasia | Dysplasia |

Hyperplasia, Hypertrophy, Dysplasia

3-48

hypo

The prefix for below or less than normal is _____.

3-49

The combining form for growth or development is **troph/o**. A/trophy means progressive degeneration. When an organ or tissue that has developed properly wastes away or decreases in size, it is undergoing

a/trophy
at' rō fē
or hypo/trophy
hī **pot'** rə fē

_____.

3-50

Atrophy or hypotrophy occurs in many tissues. When muscles are not nourished or exercised, they undergo

atrophy
hypotrophy

_____ or _____.

ANSWER COLUMN

3-51

As a result of weight lifting, body builders' muscles increase in size or overdevelop, called

hyper/trophy
hī **per'** trō fē.

_____.

3-52

crani/o is used in words referring to the crani/um or skull. Recall that -plasty is the suffix for surgical repair.

surgical repair of the
skull or cranium

Crani/o/plasty means *_____

_____.

3-53

-ectomy is a suffix meaning to cut out. The word meaning **excision** of part of the cranium (skull) is _____.

crani/ectomy
krā nē **ek'** tə mē

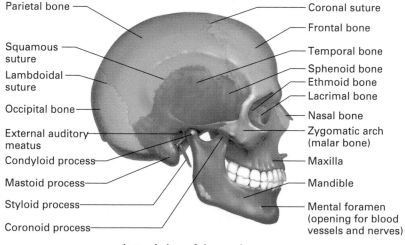

Parietal bone —
Coronal suture
Frontal bone
Squamous suture
Temporal bone
Lambdoidal suture
Sphenoid bone
Ethmoid bone
Lacrimal bone
Occipital bone
Nasal bone
External auditory meatus
Zygomatic arch (malar bone)
Condyloid process
Maxilla
Mastoid process
Mandible
Styloid process
Mental foramen (opening for blood vessels and nerves)
Coronoid process

Lateral view of the cranium

ANSWER COLUMN

3-54

The word for **incision** into the skull is

crani/otomy
krā nē **ot'** ə mē

_____.

3-55

There are cranial bones. There are also

crani/al
cranial

_____ nerves. There are grooves and

furrows called _____ fissures.

3-56

adjectival

Crani/al is the _____

(noun/adjectival) form of crani/o.

3-57

Crani/o/cerebr/al refers to the skull and the cerebr/um. The

cerebr/um is a part of the brain. Cerebr/o is used to

cerebr/um
ser' ɔ brəm,
se **rē'** brum

build words about the _____.

3-58

The cerebrum is the largest part of the brain in which thought occurs.

Humans can think. Generally speaking, other animals cannot.

Humans have a larger and better-developed

cerebrum

_____ than other animals.

3-59

The adjectival form of cerebrum is

cerebr/al
ser' ə brəl, se **rē'** bral

_____.

ANSWER COLUMN

3-60

There is a cerebral reflex. There are cerebral fissures.
You have probably heard of _____ hemorrhage.

cerebral

3-61

Cerebr/o/path/y (ser e **brop'** a thē) means *_____

any disease of the
   cerebrum or disease
   of the cerebrum

_____

_____.

3-62

Cerebr/o/malacia means *_____

softening the
   cerebrum

_____.

3-63

A cerebr/oma is a *_____

cerebral tumor or
   any mass in the brain

_____.

3-64

An incision into the cerebrum to remove an abscess is a

cerebr/o/tomy
ser ə **brot'** ə mē

_____.

3-65

Cerebr/o/vascular refers to the blood vessels of the brain. A stroke or
brain attack is caused by a blockage of blood flow to the brain that
may be caused by a thrombus or a broken blood vessel. Stroke or
brain attack is also called _____

cerebr/o/vascular
ser' ē brō **vas'** kyōō lər

accident (CVA).

ANSWER COLUMN

3-66

Cerebr/o/spin/al refers to the brain and spinal cord. There is fluid that bathes the cerebrum and spinal cord. It is

cerebr/o/spin/al
ser ē brō **spī′** nəl

_____ fluid (CSF).

3-67

A cerebr/o/spin/al puncture (also called lumbar puncture (LP) or spinal tap) is sometimes done to remove

cerebrospinal

_____ fluid.

3-68

cerebrospinal

There is a disease called _____ meningitis.

3-69

The meninges is a three-layered membrane that covers the brain and spinal cord. These three layers are the pia mater, arachnoid, and dura mater. The protective covering of the brain and spinal cord is the

mening/es
men **in′** jēz

_____.

3-70

A herniation of the membrane covering the brain and spinal cord is a _____.

mening/o/cele
men **in′** gō sēl′

ANSWER COLUMN

meninges

3-71

A meningocele is a herniation of the _____.

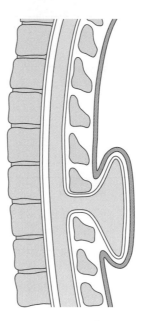

Meningocele

3-72

meninges

Mening/o/malac/ia means softening of the

_____.

3-73

mening/itis
men in **jĭ'** tis

Refer to the inside front cover for the **"g" rule**. Mening/itis can occur as cerebr/al meningitis, as spin/al meningitis, or as cerebr/o/spin/al

_____.

3-74

meningitis

There are many kinds of meningitis. The tubercle bacillus can cause tuberculous meningitis. Mening/o/cocci are bacteria that cause epidemic _____.

ANSWER COLUMN

3-75

aden/o is used in words that refer to glands. The word
root is _____. The combining form is
_____.

aden
aden/o

3-76

Build a word that means inflammation of a gland (remember the
word root + suffix rule) _____.

aden/itis
ad ən **ī'** tis

3-77

Aden/ectomy means excision or removal of a gland. The
part that means excision is _____.
The part that means gland is _____.
The word for removal of a gland is _____.

ectomy
aden
aden/ectomy
ad ən **ek'** tə mē

3-78

An adenectomy is a surgical procedure. If a gland is tumorous, part
or all of it may be excised. This operation is
an _____.

adenectomy

3-79

A tumor is an abnormal growth of cells, also termed a neoplasm.
-oma is the suffix for tumor. Form a word that
means tumor of a gland. _____.

aden/oma

3-80

When a thyroid _____ (tumor of a gland)
is found, a partial _____ (excision
of gland) may be performed.

adenoma
adenectomy or
   thyroidectomy

ANSWER COLUMN

3-81

Recall that -pathy is a suffix for disease. Aden/o/pathy means any disease of a gland. In this word you have

aden/o

a combining form _____ plus

pathy

a suffix _____ to form the word

aden/o/pathy

_____.

ad ən **op'** a thē

3-82

Metastasis is the transfer of a disease from one organ to another. Carcinoma may metastasize (spread to other parts of the body) through the bloodstream. The intestine has a rich blood supply.

carcin/oma

For this reason, intestinal _____ is extremely

kär si **nō'** ma

dangerous, as it may metastasize to the liver.

NOTE: meta- means beyond, and -stasis means in one place (staying, control, or stopping). Metastasis means spreading beyond the original place.

3-83

Carcinoma may be confined to the site (from the Greek situs) of its

carcinoma

origin. In this case, it is called _____ in situ.

3-84

Form a word that means a cancerous tumor of glandular

aden/o/carcinoma

tissue. _____.

ad' e nō kär si **nō'** ma

ANSWER COLUMN

3-85

black

melan/oma
mel ə **nō′** ma

melan/o means _____. Melan/osis means black pigmentation. A word that means black tumor is _____.

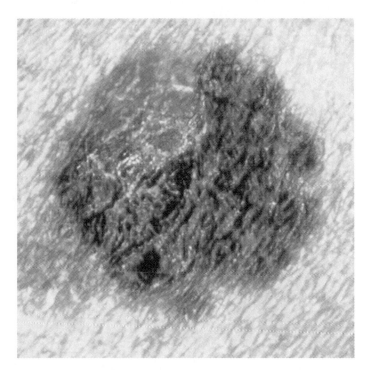

Melanoma   *Courtesy of the American Academy of Dermatology*

3-86

Melanin is the pigment that gives dark color to the hair, skin, and choroid of the eye. A black pigmented cell is a

_____.

melan/o/cyte
mel′ ə nō sīt
mə **lan′** ə sīt

ANSWER COLUMN

3-87

You have already learned that a carcin/oma is a form of cancer. A darkly pigmented cancer is

melan/o/carcin/oma
mel′ ə nō kär si **nō′** ma

_____ , also called malignant melanoma.

3-88

Whenever any hairless mole on the skin turns black and grows, a physician should be consulted, for there is possible danger of malignant melanoma, or

melanocarcinoma

_____ .

TUMOR TERMINOLOGY
Epithelial Tissue

Combining Form	Meaning	Term
Benign	_Noncancerous_	
aden/o	gland	adenoma
melan/o	dark pigmented	melanoma
papillo/o	small elevation	papilloma
fibr/o	fibrous tissue	adenofibroma
Malignant	_Cancerous_	carcinoma
aden/o	gland, glandular tissue	adenocarcinoma
melan/o	dark pigmented	melanocarcinoma (malignant melanoma) squamous cell carcinoma basal cell carcinoma
Benign		
oste/o	bone	osteoma
chondr/o	cartilage	chondroma
leiomy/o	smooth muscle	leiomyoma
lip/o	fat	lipoma
ather/o	fatty, porridgelike	atheroma
hem/angi/o	blood vessel	hemangioma
neur/o	nerve	neuroma

ANSWER COLUMN

TUMOR TERMINOLOGY
Epithelial Tissue

Combining Form	Meaning	Term
Malignant		
oste/o	bone	osteosarcoma
chondr/o	cartilage	chondrosarcoma
leiomy/o	smooth muscle	leiomyosarcoma
lip/o	fat	liposarcoma
angi/o	vessel	angiosarcoma
leuk/o	white	leukemia
myel/o	bone marrow	myeloma
lymph/o	lymphatic	lymphosarcoma
neur/o	nerve	neurosarcoma
rhabd/o/my/o	rod shaped, muscle	rhabdomyosarcoma

3-89

adenitis
adenectomy

When a gland is found to have a mild inflammation or
_____, no _____ (surgery) is
indicated.

3-90

tumor
fat

An adenoma is a glandular tumor -oma is the suffix for
_____. A lip/oma is a tumor containing fat.
Lip/o is the word root–combining form for _____.

3-91

lip/oma
li **pō'** ma

A lip/oma is usually benign (noncancerous). A fat tumor
is called a _____.

3-92

cancerous tumor or
malignant tumor

carcin/o is the combining form for cancer. A carcin/oma
is a *_____
_____.

ANSWER COLUMN

3-93

A carcinoma may occur in almost any part of the body composed of epithelial tissue. A stomach cancer is called

carcinoma

gastric _____.

3-94

onc/o is a combining form meaning tumor. The study of tumors is onc/o/logy. A specialist in the study of tumors

onc/o/logist
on **kol'** ō jist

is called an _____.

3-95

A hospitalized patient with a disease caused by a tumor

onc/o/logy
on **kol'** ō je

would be treated on the _____ unit.

3-96

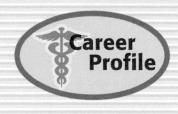

Career
Profile

Radiation therapists (RT[T]) are specialists in the administration of radiation therapy for the purpose of treating cancer. They begin their careers as registered radiographic technologists (RT[R]) and through advanced study become certified to administer radiation treatments. They work closely with radiologists, who are physicians specialized in the use of radiation for diagnosis and treatment, as well as oncologists, who are experts in the diagnosis and treatment of tumor disorders. The department in which they work is called Radiation Oncology.

3-97

ather/o is the combining form for fatty or porridgelike. A tumorlike thickening and degeneration of the blood vessel walls that is caused by fatty deposits is called an

ather/oma
ath er **ō'** ma

_____.

A fatty deposit causing hardening of the blood vessels is

ather/o/scler/osis
ath' er ō skler **ō'** sis

_____.

ANSWER COLUMN

3-98

resembling

muc

muc/o

Muc/oid means resembling mucus. -oid is a suffix meaning _____. The word root for mucus is _____, and its combining form is _____.

3-99

muc/oid

myōō' koid

Mucoid is an adjective that means resembling or like mucus. There is a substance in connective tissue that resembles mucus. This is a _____ substance.

3-100

lip/o

lip/oid

lip' oid

The combining form for fat is _____ -oid is a suffix that means like or resembling. Build a word that means fatlike or resembling fat: _____.

3-101

lipoid

In proper amounts, cholesterol is essential to health, but too much may cause atherosclerosis. Cholesterol is an alcohol that resembles fat; therefore, it is _____.

3-102

muc/us

myōō' kus

Muc/us is a secretion of the muc/ous membrane. -us is a noun suffix. -ous is an adjectival suffix. The muc/ous membrane secretes _____.

3-103

mucus

Mucus is secreted by cells in the nose. It traps dust and bacteria from the air. One of the body's protective devices is _____.

ANSWER COLUMN

3-104

The tissue that secretes mucus is the

muc/ous
myōō′ kus

_____ membrane or muc/osa.

3-105

The mucous membrane or mucosa is found lining the body openings. This protective, mucous membrane also

muc/osa
myōō **kō′** sa

can be called the _____.

3-106

mucus
mucoid

The intestinal mucosa secretes _____. Anything that
resembles mucus is _____. Mucoid substances are
not mucus; therefore, they are not secreted by

mucosa or
   mucous membrane

the *_____.

3-107

The serous membranes line the closed body cavities and cover the
outside of organs such as the intestines. **Serosa** is the noun form.

ser/osa
sē **ro′** sa

The intestinal _____ is a membrane that covers
the intestine.

3-108

ser/ous
sēr′ us

The mucous membranes line the open body cavities, and
the _____ (adjective) membranes line the
closed cavities.

3-109

my/o is the combining form for muscle. A spasm of a nerve is a
neur/o/spasm. A spasm of a muscle is a

my/o/spasm
mī′ ō spazm

_____.

ANSWER COLUMN

3-110

Neuralgia is nerve pain. Neuropathy is a disease of the

nerves

_____.

3-111

Neurology is the medical specialty that deals with the nervous system. One who specializes in diagnosis and treatment of diseases of the nervous system is a

neur/o/logist

noo **rol′** ə jist

_____.

Refer to the illustration of the nerves below.

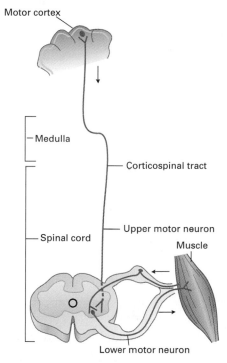

Motor cortex

Medulla

Corticospinal tract

Upper motor neuron

Muscle

Spinal cord

Lower motor neuron

Motor pathways of the CNS

ANSWER COLUMN

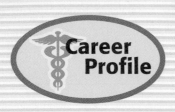
Career Profile

3-112

If a disease of the nervous system requires surgery, the **neurologist** will refer the patient to another physician called a **neurosurgeon**. The **neurosurgeon** requires 14 years of careful study and training to be able to perform the delicate skill of surgery on the brain, spinal cord, and other nerve tissue structures.

3-113

Build a word meaning:
inflammation of a nerve

neur/itis
noo **rī** tis

_____;

destruction of nerve tissue

neur/o/lysis
noo' **rol'** a sis

_____;

surgical repair of nerves

neur/o/plasty
noo' rō plas tē

_____;

nervous system surgeon

neur/o/surgeon
noo rō **sur'** jən

_____.

3-114

The combining form that refers to tissue is **hist/o**. Hist/o/lysis is the destruction of _____.

tissue

3-115

A hist/o/genous substance is a substance that is made by _____.

tissue

ANSWER COLUMN

3-116

Build a word meaning:
the study of tissue

hist/o/logy
his **tol'** ə je

_____;

one who studies tissues

hist/o/log/ist
his **tol'** ə jist

_____.

3-117

Build a word meaning:
an embryonic tissue (cell)

hist/o/blast

_____;

a tissue cell

hist/o/cyte

_____;

resembling tissue

hist/oid
(You pronounce)

_____.

3-118

ne/o in words means new. Ne/o/genesis means generation

new

of _____ tissue.

3-119

new
new

Ne/o/nat/al refers to the _____ born. A
ne/o/plasm is a tumor or _____ growth
(formation—plasm/o).

3-120

A special unit for the newborn is the

ne/o/natal
nē ō **nāt'** əl

_____ intensive care unit.

ANSWER COLUMN

3-121

Ne/o/plasm refers to any kind of tumor or abnormal growth of cells.
A nonmalignant tumor is called a benign

ne/o/plasm
nē′ ō plaz əm

_____.

3-122

A neoplasm may also be a malignant tumor. Recall that

malignant neoplasm
neoplasm
neoplasm

carcinoma is a *_____. A melanoma
is also a _____. A melanocarcinoma
is a malignant _____.

3-123

neoplasm

A sarcoma is also a malignant _____
of connective tissue.

3-124

Build a word meaning:
any new disease

ne/o/pathy

_____;

abnormal fear of new things

ne/o/phobia
(You pronounce)

_____.

3-125

Recall that anti- is a prefix meaning against. A therapeutic agent that
works against neoplasms is called an

anti/ne/o/plas/tic
an′ ti nē′ ō **plas′** tik

_____ plast ic ___ agent.

ANSWER COLUMN

3-126

Rhabd/o is a combining form of Greek origin that means rod-shaped. It may be found in words about rod-shaped parasites, like the nematode worm *Rhabditoidea*. If you see the combining form **rhabd/o**, think of _____.

rod-shaped

3-127

Recall that a blast is an immature cell. A my/o/blast is an immature muscle cell. A rhabd/o/my/o/blast is an abnormal immature muscle cell that may lead to the development of sarcoma. Use your dictionary to analyze the meaning of these terms and their correct pronunciation.
rhabdomyoma

rhabd/o/my/oma
rab′ dō mī **ō′** mə
rhabd/o/my/o/sarc/oma
rab′ dȯ mī′ ō sär **kō′** mə

** _____

rhabdomyosarcoma
** _____.

That's great! You are really getting good at working with some very complex terms.

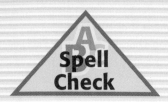

3-128

Notice the unusual spelling of the combining form **rhabdo**. The "rh" is Greek in origin. The "h" is silent, but don't forget to put it in. You will be learning many more word parts with an "rh" spelling in Unit 4. When you see them you will know that the "h" is silent.

The following medical abbreviations correspond to the terms in Unit 3.

Abbreviation	Meaning
ASCP (MT)	American Society of Clinical Pathology (medical technologist)
Ca, CA	cancer
CIS	carcinoma in situ
CNS	central nervous system
CSF	cerebrospinal fluid
CVA	cerebrovascular accident (stroke)
EEG	electroencephalogram
END	electroneurodiagnostic (technologist)
IPV	inactivated polio vaccine
LP	lumbar puncture
met., metas., mets.	metastasis
MRI	magnetic resonance imaging
RT(N)	radiologic technologist (nuclear)
RT(R)	radiographic technologist (registered)
RT(T)	radiographic technologist (radiation therapy)

You have been introduced to many new terms in this unit. To make sure you know them well, work the review exercises on the following pages. Also, listen to the audio CD-ROM accompanying the third edition of *Medical Terminology Made Easy,* and practice pronunciation.

UNIT 3
REVIEW EXERCISE

Part 1: Review the terms you have learned in this unit by drawing the diagonal lines between the word parts and writing the meaning of each term. Use your medical dictionary or the frames if you need help. After you have completed these tasks, say each term aloud to practice pronunciation.

1. adenectomy _____

2. adenitis _____

3. adenocarcinoma _____

4. antineoplastic _____

5. atheroma _____

6. atherosclerosis _____

7. carcinoma _____

8. cephalalgia _____

9. cephalic _____

10. cerebroma _____

11. cerebromalacia _____

12. cerebrospinal _____

13. craniectomy _____

14. cranioplasty _____

15. electroencephalogram _____

16. electroneurodiagnostic _____

17. encephalitis _____

18. encephalocele _____

19. encephaloma _____

20. encephalomeningitis _____

21. encephalotomy _____

22. histology _____

23. hydrocephalus _____

24. lipoma _____

25. melanocarcinoma _____

26. meningocele _____

27. myelocytic _____

UNIT 3
REVIEW EXERCISE

28. myelodysplasia _____

29. myelopathy _____

30. myospasm _____

31. neonatal _____

32. neogenesis _____

33. neoplasm _____

34. neurology _____

35. neurosurgeon _____

36. oncologist _____

37. poliomyelitis _____

38. psychiatrist _____

39. rhabdomyosarcoma _____

40. sarcoma _____

41. visceral _____

42. viscerogenic _____

Part 2: Match each term with its correct meaning.

_____ 1. cephalalgia

_____ 2. hydrocephalus

_____ 3. craniotomy

_____ 4. meningitis

_____ 5. myelodysplasia

_____ 6. encephalocele

_____ 7. hypotrophy

_____ 8. cerebropathy

_____ 9. adenopathy

_____ 10. cerebrospinal

a. lack of development

b. herniation of the meninges

c. herniation of the colon

d. headache

e. defective development

f. herniation of the brain

g. enlarged head caused by fluid in the brain

h. defective development of the spinal cord

i. inflammation of the brain

j. general term for brain disease (cerebrum)

k. incision into the skull

l. pertaining to the brain and spinal cord

m. softening of the bones

n. inflammation of the membrane surrounding the spinal cord

o. disease of a gland

UNIT 3
REVIEW EXERCISE

Part 3: Write the medical term that means:

1. inflammation of a gland _____

2. cancer of a dark pigmented tissue _____

3. excision of a gland _____

4. the study of the nervous system_____

5. a physician specializing in neoplasms_____

6. pertaining to organs _____

7. an agent that works against tumors _____

8. resembling fat _____   _____

9. surgical repair of the skull_____

Part 4: Use the medical terms listed below to complete these sentences:

neurologist	electroencephalography	melanocytes
encephalomalacia	osteosarcoma	psychiatrist
hypertrophy	histolysis	leiomyoma
lymphadenoma	cranial	neurosurgeon
peritoneum	cephalic	serosa
myelocele		

1. The _____ ordered an EEG on a patient suspected of having a seizure disorder due to brain damage.

2. Part of the spinal cord was protruding through a vertebra in this patient with a _____.

3. _____ was caused by a bacteria that destroys human tissue.

4. A 45-year-old female patient complained of lower abdominal pain and excessive vaginal bleeding during her menses. Upon examination, a benign _____ (or fibroid) was discovered in the uterine musculature.

5. It was noted that the baby was born head first. This is called a _____ presentation.

6. "I'm only afraid when I have to try new things," said Mr. P. A. Noya. He may have been suffering from _____.

7. After two months of weight training, George noticed _____ of his leg muscles.

UNIT 3
REVIEW EXERCISE

8. Ms. Melanie Oma admires her brown skin after a day at the beach. She can thank her
   _____ for creating dark pigment to help protect her skin from the sun's
   ultraviolet rays.

9. Following a suicide attempt, the young man was admitted to the psychiatric unit for treatment by
   a _____.

Part 5: Draw a line to match the abbreviation with its meaning.

1. Ca   metastasis

2. RT(T)   electroencephalogram

3. metas   central nervous system

4. EEG   American Society of Clinical Pathology

5. ASCP   inactivated polio vaccine

6. CNS   Radiologic Technologist (Radiation Therapy)

7. IPV   cancer

**UNIT 3
REVIEW EXERCISE**

Part 6: Label the following structures of the head and neck. Then draw a line to the matching combining form for that structure.

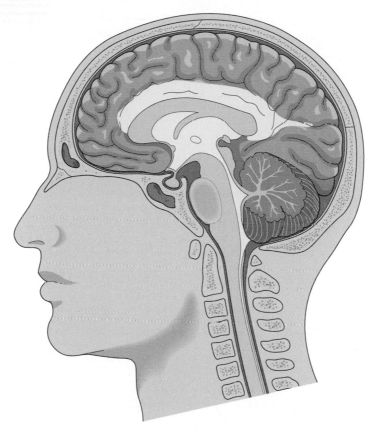

Structures of the Head and Neck

myel/o _____

crani/o _____

mening/o _____

cerebr/o _____

encephal/o _____

cephal/o _____

Unit 3 Puzzle

As a self-test work the crossword puzzle and then check your answers in Appendix F.

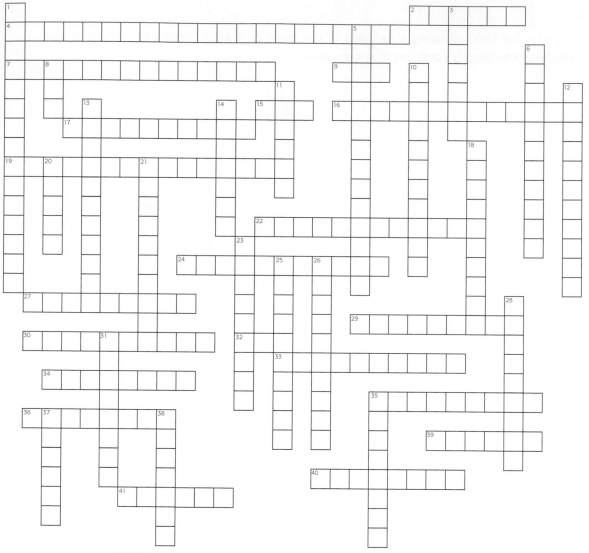

ACROSS

2. resembling mucus
4. brain wave measurement instrument
7. brain disease
9. radiographic technologist (registered)
15. electroencephalogram (abbrev.)
16. brain herniation
17. dark pigmented cell
19. fatty deposit causing hardening of arteries
22. operates on the nervous system
24. too much growth
27. study of tissues
29. poor or defective development
30. destruction of nerve tissue
32. radiation therapist (abbrev.)
33. tumor specialist
34. pertaining to organs
35. bad or cancerous
36. new growth
39. fat tumor
40. the wall of an organ
41. pertaining to mucus

DOWN

1. pertaining to the vessels of the brain
3. pertaining to the skull
5. agent against cancer
6. overdevelopment in size
8. central nervous system (abbrev.)
10. headache
11. membrane lining closed cavities (noun)
12. herniation of the membrane around the spine
13. physician of the nervous system
14. progressive degeneration
18. inflammation of the meninges
20. used to mean water
21. incision into the skull
23. tumor of the cerebrum
25. abdominal membrane
26. excision of a gland
28. cancer of epithelial-type tissue
31. the study of tumors and abnormal growths
35. inflammation of the spinal cord
37. vomiting
38. suffix for softening

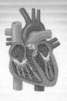

UNIT 4
Digestive System

The following word parts are introduced in this unit. Study these words, parts, meanings, and examples. Then proceed to the first frame. Remember, you are using a word-building system, so return to the previous units to review old terms.

COMBINING FORMS

chol/e (gall, bile)
cholecyst/o (gallbladder)
col/o (colon)
cyst/o (bladder, sac)
duoden/o (duodenum)
enter/o (intestine)
esophag/o (esophagus)
esthesi/o (sensation)
gastr/o (stomach)
gingiv/o (gums)
gloss/o, lingu/o (tongue)
hepat/o (liver)
lith/o (stone, calculus)
pancreat/o (pancreas)
peps/o (digestion)
phag/o (eat, swallow)
phor/o (bear, carry)
proct/o (anus and rectum)
rect/o (rectum)
sigmoid/o (sigmoid colon)
splen/o (spleen)
stomat/o (mouth)
trich/o (hair)

PREFIXES

dys- (difficult, painful, bad, abnormal)
eu- (easy, good)
mal- (bad, poor)
sub- (below)

SUFFIXES

-cele (hernia)
-centesis (surgical puncture)
-ectomy (excise)
-iasis (condition, usually infestation)
-meter (instrument), -metry (process)
 (measuring)
-ostomy (make a new opening)
-pepsia (digestion)
-phagia (eat, swallow)
-plegia (paralysis)
-rrhagia (hemorrhage)
-rrhaphy (suture)
-rrhea (flow, discharge)
-rrhexis (rupture)
-scope (instrument used to look)
-scopy (process of looking using a scope)
-tomy (cut into)
-tripsy (surgical crushing)

Word Examples

COMBINING FORMS

cholelith
cholecystogram
colectomy
cystitis
duodenotomy
gastroenterology
esophagitis
hyperesthesia
gastrectomy
gingivoplasty
glossal
hepatorrhagia
lithiasis
pancreatolysis
peptic
phagocyte
dysphoria
proctoplegia
rectorrhaphy
sigmoidoscope
splenomegaly
stomatitis
trichophagia

PREFIXES

dysphagia
euphoria
malnutrition
sublingual

SUFFIXES

rectocele
abdominocentesis
hepatectomy
cholelithiasis
esthesiometer
pelvimetry
colostomy
dyspepsia
bradyphagia
glossoplegia
gastrorrhagia
cystorrhaphy
stomatorrhea
colorrhexis
enteroscope
colonoscopy
duodenostomy
gastrotomy
lithotripsy

ANSWER COLUMN

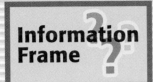

Information Frame

4-1

The digestive system is like a long tube that starts at the mouth and ends at the anus. It has three basic layers: a mucous membrane inner lining, a middle layer composed of smooth muscle, and an outer layer of serous membrane. Along the way there are specialized structures, such as the esophagus, stomach, and intestines, which each have an important function in moving food through the system, breaking it down, absorbing the nutrients, and eliminating solid waste (feces).

4-2

mucous
muscle
membrane

The inner lining of the digestive system is made of
_____ membrane; the middle layer is
smooth _____; and the outer layer is
a serous _____.

4-3

feces
fē′sēz

The solid waste that is eliminated is called
_____ or stool.

4-4

stomat/algia
stō mə **tal′** jē ə

"Stoma" is the Greek word for mouth. **Stomat/o** is the combining form for mouth. Form a word meaning: pain in the mouth
_____.

4-5

inflammation of
   the mouth

Stomat/itis means

*_____.

surgical repair of
   the mouth

Stomat/o/plasty means

*_____.

ANSWER COLUMN

4-6

-scope is a suffix for an instrument used to examine.
A micr/o/scope is an instrument for examining something small.

stomat/o/scope
stō **mat'** ō skōp
stomat/o/scopy
stō mə **tos'** kə pē

An instrument for examining the mouth is a _____.
The process of examining with this instrument
is _____.

4-7

The combining form for tongue is **gloss/o**.

inflammation of
  the tongue
excision of
  the tongue

Gloss/itis means *_____
_____.

Gloss/ectomy means *_____
_____.

4-8

Using the word root, build a word meaning: pain in the tongue

gloss/algia
glos **al'** jē a
gloss/al
glos' əl

_____;

pertaining to the tongue

_____ al .

4-9

Information Frame ??

Tubelike structures have many things in common when they develop problems, whether they are part of the digestive system or the cardiovascular system. Study this table of conditions:

Condition	Description	Example
atresia	congenital closure of a tubular organ	biliary atresia
occlusion	act of being closed	coronary occlusion
stenosis	narrowing or stricture	pyloric stenosis
stricture	decrease in the diameter of a tube	spasmodic stricture
collapse	abnormal falling in of walls of a structure	circulatory collapse
intussusception	prolapse of one part into another	ileocecal intussusception

Look at the diagram of the digestive system and study the structures.

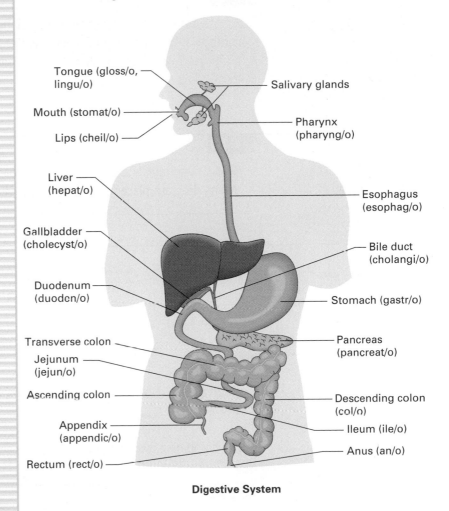

Digestive System

4-10

hypo- is a prefix meaning below or under. Cranial nerve 12 is the hypo/gloss/al nerve. It supplies nerve impulses
*_____. A structure that is located under the tongue is

_____.

under the tongue or
   to the tongue
hypo/gloss/al
hī pō **glos′** al

NOTE: **sub** and **lingual** are Latin word parts. **hypo** and **glossal** are Greek word parts. Generally, original languages are not mixed as they form words.

ANSWER COLUMN

4-11

sub- is a prefix that means the same as hypo-. **lingu/o** is another combining form for tongue. Lingual is the adjectival form. sub- is a prefix used with **lingu/o**. A medication administered under the tongue is a _____ medication.

sub/lingu/al
sub **ling'** gwal

4-12

Nitroglycerin tablets are administered sublingually. This means they are placed * _____

under the tongue

_____.

4-13

Two words you have learned that mean under the tongue are:

hyp/o/gloss/al
sub/lingu/al

_____;

_____.

4-14

gingiv/o is the combining form for gums. Gingiv/al means * _____.

pertaining to
   the gums
gingiv/o

The combining form for gums is _____.

4-15

Build a word meaning:
inflammation of the gums

gingiv/itis
jin ji **vī'** tis

_____;

gum pain

gingiv/algia
jin ji **val'** jē ə

_____.

ANSWER COLUMN

4-16

The word esophagus is built from "phago," meaning eat. **esophag/o** is used in words about the esophagus. The

esophag/eal   adjective is _____ eal.

                       word root   suffix

4-17

Build an adjective meaning pertaining to the esophagus and stomach.

esophag/o/gastr/ic   _____ gastr   ic

                       or
gastr/o/esophag/eal   gastr   o _____
(You pronounce)

4-18

gastr is the word root for stomach.

algia   One suffix for pain is _____.
gastr/algia   Stomach pain is _____.
gas **tral'** jē ə

4-19

The Greek word **"tomos"** means cutting. From this word we build many suffixes that refer to cutting including: -ectomy, -tomy, -tome, and -ostomy.

The common word root found in all of these is

tom/   _____.

ANSWER COLUMN

4-20

Study this table of suffixes and then complete the statements following:

Suffix	Meaning	Example
-tome	cutting instrument	derm/a/tome
-tomy	to cut into (incise)	crani/o/tomy
-ectomy	to cut out (excise)	gastr/ectomy
-stomy	to form a new opening (surgically)	col/o/stomy

4-21

Use the word root for stomach to create surgical terms that mean:
incision into the stomach

gastr/o/tomy
gas **tro'** tō mē

_____;

gastr/ectomy
gas **trek'** tō mē

removal of the stomach

_____;

form an opening in the stomach, as through the abdomen for feeding someone who cannot swallow

gastr/o/stomy
gas **tros'** tō mē

_____.

4-22

Gastr/ectomy means excision (removal) of all or part of the stomach.

excision or
removal

-ectomy is a suffix meaning _____.

4-23

Gastr/o/rrhagia means stomach hemorrhage. Encephal/o/rrhagia

hem/o/rrhage
hem' ə rəj

means brain _____.

ANSWER COLUMN

4-24

There are four Greek origin suffixes that have a very unusual spelling. They all contain **"rrh."** Look at this table and then use this information when building words with these suffixes.

Suffix	Meaning	Example/Pronunciation
-rrhea	discharge, flow	dia/rrhea dī ə rē′ ə
-rrhagia	bleeding, hemorrhage	gastr/o/rrhagia gas trō **rā′** jē ə
-rrhaphy	suturing, stitching	rect/o/rrhaphy rek **tôr′** ə fē
-rrhexis	rupture	enter/o/rrhexis en′ ter ō **rek′** sis

4-25

Spell Check

"rrh" is pronounced like **"r"** as in rage, raft, and Rex. Make sure you include the **"rrh"** in the spelling of the suffixes listed above even though the second **"r"** and the **"h"** are silent.

4-26

-rrhagia is the suffix for hemorrhage.

Gastr/o/rrhagia means *_____.

Gastr/itis means *_____.

Gastr/ic means *_____.

stomach hemorrhage
inflammation of
   the stomach
pertaining to the stomach

4-27

enter/o is used in words about the small intestine or the intestine in general. Tablets that dissolve in the intestine may have been treated with an **enteric** coating. Inflammation of the intestine is

_____.

enter/itis
en ter **ī′** tis

ANSWER COLUMN

4-28

The internal medicine specialty that studies diseases of the stomach and intestine is:

gastr/o/enter/o/logy
gas′ trō en ter **ol′** ə jē

_____.

4-29

Recall the prefix dys- meaning difficulty or pain. Dysentery is a disorder of the intestine characterized by inflammation, pain, and diarrhea. When caused by an amoeba-type parasite, it is called amoebic

dys/enter/y
dis′ en ter ē

_____.

4-30

Form a word meaning:
pertaining to the stomach and small intestine

gastr/o/enter/ic
gas′ trō en **ter′** ik

_____;

hemorrhage of the small intestine

enter/o/rrhagia
en′ ter ō **rā′** jē ə

_____.

4-31

Recall -cele is a suffix meaning hernia. Build a word meaning:
intestinal hernia

enter/o/cele
en′ ter ō sēl

_____.

4-32

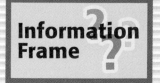
Information Frame

Here's another free frame for those interested in -stomy.
mouth—opening   stoma—mouth
y   noun ending (process)
make a **mouth** (opening) by cutting—stomy

ANSWER COLUMN

4-33

Gastr/o/duoden/o/stomy means forming a new opening between the stomach and duodenum. A surgeon who removes the natural connection between the duodenum and stomach and then forms a new connection is doing a

gastr/o/duoden/o/stomy
gas′ trō dōo′ ō də **nos′** tə mē

_____.

4-34

A gastroduodenostomy is a surgical procedure. When the pyloric sphincter, a valve that controls the amount of food going from the stomach to the duodenum, no longer functions, a

gastroduodenostomy

_____ may be done.

4-35

When a portion of the first part of the small intestine is removed because of cancer, a new opening is formed by performing a

gastroduodenostomy
or
duodenostomy

_____.

4-36

-tomy is a combining form you may use as a suffix because it connects directly to a combining form. A duoden/o/tomy is an incision into the _____.

duodenum

4-37

If a duoden/o/tomy is an incision into the duodenum, the word part meaning **incision** is _____.

-tomy

4-38

-tomy means incision into. An incision into the duodenum is a

duoden/o/tomy
dōo ō də **not′** ə mē

_____.

ANSWER COLUMN

4-39

Recall that -stomy means making a new opening.
The word to form a new opening into the duodenum is

duoden/ostomy
dōō' ō dən **os'** tə mē

_____.

4-40

A duodenostomy can be formed in more than one manner.
If it is formed with the stomach, it is called a

gastr/o/duoden/ostomy
gas' trō dōō' ō den **os'** tə mē

_____.

4-41

-ostomy

The suffix for forming a new opening is _____.

4-42

col/o is the combining form for colon (large intestine).

pertaining to the
colon or large
intestine

Col/ic means *_____
_____.

inflammation of the
colon or large
intestine

Col/itis means *_____
_____.

4-43

Due to excision of part of the colon or colon disease, it may be
necessary to create an opening (stoma) into the colon from the
abdominal wall through which fecal matter passes into a bag.

col/o/stomy
ko **los'** tə mē

This procedure is called a _____.

ANSWER COLUMN

4-44

enter/o is the combining form for small intestine. The
adjectival form is _____ ic .

enteric
en **ter'** ik

enter/itis
en ter ī' tis

enter/o/scope
en' ter ō skōp

Inflammation of the small intestine is _____.
An instrument to examine the small intestine is the

_____.

4-45

The combining form for rectum is **rect/o**.
Rect/al means *_____.

pertaining to the
    rectum

a rectal hernia or
    hernia of the rectum

A rect/o/cele is *_____

_____.

4-46

Recall that -scope refers to an instrument used to look with. Build a
word meaning:
instrument for examining the rectum

rect/o/scope
rek' tō skōp

_____.

4-47

Hem/o/rrhoids are caused by dilatation of veins that usually develop
in the rectum. Increased pressure due to straining during bowel
movements, childbirth, or trauma may cause

hemorrhoids
hem' ō roidz

_____.

ANSWER COLUMN

4-48

Treatment of hemorrhoids may include surgical removal or

hemorrhoid/ectomy
hem′ ō roid **ek′** tō mē

_____.

4-49

Spell Check

Once again, you have a term from Greek origin including an "rrh" in its spelling. Hemorrhoid and hemorrhage are very similar. Remember to use the "rrh" in spelling, but do not pronounce the second "r" or the "h."

4-50

-scopy refers to the process of using a scope. The process of examining the rectum with a rectoscope

rect/o/scopy
rek **tos′** kō pē
rect/o/scopic
rek tō **skop′** ik

is called _____. In doing this, the physician has performed a

_____ examination.

        (adjective)

4-51

Information Frame ???

A more common procedure is a **sigmoid/o/scopy**. This is done using a sigmoidoscope introduced through the sigmoid colon to the large intestine.

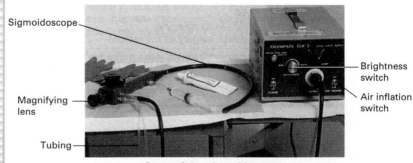

Parts of the sigmoidoscope

ANSWER COLUMN

4-52

Colon cancer, or adenocarcinoma of the colon, is one of the most common forms of cancer in men and women. Early detection and treatment can increase the chance for recovery. The procedure used to look at the sigmoid colon with a scope is called

sigmoid/o/scopy
sig' moid **os'** kō pē

_____.

4-53

colon/o may also be used to build words about the colon. Colon/o/scopy is a procedure that uses a long flexible illuminated scope to examine the rectum, sigmoid, and descending, transverse, and ascending colon. A complete exam of the colon using a scope is a

colon/o/scopy
kō' lən **os'** kō pē

_____.

4-54

-rrhaphy is a suffix meaning suturing. Build a word meaning:
plastic surgery of the rectum

rect/o/plasty
rek' tō plas tē

_____;

suturing (stitching) of the rectum

rect/o/rrhaphy
rek **tôr'** ə fē

_____.

4-55

proct/o is the combining form for the rectal area. A
proct/o/log/ist is one who *_____

specializes in diseases
   of the rectal area
   (anus and rectum)

_____.

study of diseases
   of rectum area
   (anus and rectum)

Proct/o/logy is *_____

_____

ANSWER COLUMN

4-56

-plegia is a suffix meaning paralysis. Build a word meaning:
paralysis of the anus and rectum

proct/o/plegia
prok tō **plē′** jē ə

_____.

4-57

A proctologist examines the rectum with a

proct/o/scope
prok′ tō skōp

_____.

This examination is called

proct/o/scopy
prok **tos′** kə pē

_____.

4-58

Recall that -rrhaphy is a suffix meaning suturing. Build a word
meaning:
suturing of the rectum and anus

proct/o/rrhaphy
prok **tôr′** ə fē

_____.

4-59

hepat/o is the combining form for liver. It comes from the Greek
word "hepar," meaning liver. Hepat/ic means

pertaining to
   the liver

*_____.

Hepatomegaly means

enlargement of
   the liver

*_____.

ANSWER COLUMN

4-60

Build a word meaning:
process of using a scope to examine the liver

_____;

hepat/o/scopy
hep ə **tos'** kə pē

any disease of the liver

_____.

hepat/o/pathy
hep ə **top'** ə thē

4-61

Build a word meaning:
incision into the liver

_____;

hepat/o/tomy
hep ə **tot'** ə mē

excision of (part of) the liver

_____.

hepat/ectomy
hep ə **tek'** tə mē

4-62

pancreat/o is used in words about the pancreas. Pancreat/ic means
*_____.

pertaining to the
　pancreas
destruction of
　pancreatic tissue

Pancreat/o/lysis means *_____
_____.

4-63

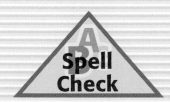

Watch the spelling! You may be tempted to put an "e" on the end of pancreas. Pancreas is the organ, and pancre*ase* is an enzyme.

ANSWER COLUMN

4-64

-lith is used as a suffix for stone or calculus. Build a word meaning:
a stone or calculus in the pancreas

pancreat/o/lith
pan′ krē **at′** ō lith

_____;

any pancreatic disease

pancreat/o/pathy
pan′ krē ə **top′** ə thē

_____.

4-65

Build a word meaning:
excision of part or all of the pancreas

pancreat/ectomy
pan′ krē ə **tek′** tə mē

_____;

incision into the pancreas

pancreat/otomy
pan′ krē ə **tot′** ə mē

_____.

4-66

Build a word meaning:

hepat/o/rrhagia
hep ə tō **rāj′** ē ə

hemorrhage of liver _____;

hepat/o/rrhaphy
hep ə **tôr′** ə fē

suture of liver   _____.

4-67

Build a word meaning:

hepat/o/cele
hep **at′** ō sēl

hernia of the liver _____;

hepat/o/lith
hep′ ə tō lith

stone in the liver _____.

ANSWER COLUMN	

4-68

splen/o is used in words about the spleen. Build a word meaning:
excision of the spleen

splen/ectomy
splē **nek'** tə mē

_____;

enlargement of the spleen

splen/o/megaly
splē nō **meg'** ə lē

_____.

4-69

Watch the spelling! "Spleen" is spelled with two "e"s, and splen/o is spelled with one.

4-70

Build a word meaning:
any disease of the spleen

splen/o/pathy
sple' **nop'** ə thē

_____;

suture of the spleen

splen/o/rrhaphy
sple' **nôr'** ə fē

_____;

hemorrhage from the spleen

splen/o/rrhagia
sple' nō **rā'** jē ə

_____.

4-71

The spleen is one of the blood-forming organs.

pain in the spleen

Splen/algia means *_____

_____.

ANSWER COLUMN

4-72

Splen/ic means

pertaining to
 the spleen

*_____

_____.

4-73

Recall the suffix -stomy. **Anastomosis** is a surgical connection between tubular structures. This word comes from "stoma," meaning mouth or opening. When an entire gastrectomy is performed, a new connection is made between the esophagus and the duodenum. This operation can also be called an

esophag/o/duoden/o/stomy
e sof′ ə gō dōō′ ə
 də **nos′** tə mē

_____ and

it is an anastomosis.

4-74

Here's a challenge! Build a word that means examination of the esophagus, stomach, and duodenum using scope: (Abbreviation: EGD.)

esophag/o/gastr/o/
 duoden/o/scopy
i sof′ ə gō gas′ trō
dōō′ ō den **os′** kō pē

_____

4-75

abdomin/o is used to form words about the abdomen. When you see abdomin/o anywhere in a word, you think

abdomen
ab′ də men
ab **dō′** men

about the _____.

4-76

Watch the spelling! Notice that the noun for abdomen is spelled with an "e" and the combining form is spelled with an "i": **abdomin/o**.

Spell
Check

ANSWER COLUMN

4-77

pertaining to the
  abdomen

Abdomin/al is an adjective that means *_____

_____.

4-78

Look up the word **para/centesis** in your dictionary. Write the definition here.

The insertion of a needle
  into a body cavity for the
  purpose of aspirating
  fluid (usually in the
  abdomen or chest).

*_____

_____.

4-79

Abdomin/o/centesis means tapping or surgical puncture of the abdomen to remove fluid or blood. The word for surgical puncture of the abdomen is

abdomin/o/centesis
ab dom′ i nō sen **tē′** sis

_____.

4-80

Centesis (surgical puncture) is a word itself. Build a word meaning surgical puncture, or insertion of a needle into a body cavity to remove fluid.

para/centesis
per ə sen **tē′** sis

_____.

4-81

amni/o refers to the amnion, the protective sac that surrounds the fetus. Tapping or puncturing this sac to remove cells for genetic testing is called

amni/o/centesis
am′ nē ō sen **tē′** sis

_____.

ANSWER COLUMN

4-82

The word for surgical puncture of the heart is

cardi/o/centesis
kär' dē ō sen **tē'** sis

_____.

4-83

lith/o is the combining form for stone or calculus. Lith/o/logy is the science of dealing with or studying

calculi
    or stones

* _____.

4-84

-genesis is used as a noun suffix meaning generating, producing, or forming. "Lithogenesis" means producing

calculi (calculus)
    or stones
litho/genic
lith ō **jen'** ik

or forming *_____.
The adjectival form of "lithogenesis" is

_____.

4-85

Using what is necessary from **lith/o**, build a word meaning an incision for the removal of a stone.

lith/o/tomy
lith **ot'** ə mē

_____.

lith/o/meter
lith **om'** ə ter

Name an instrument for measuring size of calculi.

_____.

4-86

Calculi, or stones, can be formed in many places in the body. A chol/e/lith means a gallstone. **Chol/e** is the combining

gall or bile

form for *_____.

ANSWER COLUMN

4-87

Chol/e/lith means gallstone. One result of gallbladder disease is the presence of a gallstone, or

chol/e/lith
kō' lē lith
pancreat/o/lith
pan krē **at'** ō lith

_____.

The stone in the pancreas is a

_____.

4-88

Neur/o/tripsy means the surgical crushing of a nerve. The suffix for crushing (usually by rubbing or grinding) is

–tripsy

_____.

4-89

"Tripsis," from which we get -tripsy, is a Greek word that means rub or massage. Tripsis can be carried to the point of crushing or grinding. Surgical crushing of a

neur/o/tripsy
noo' rō trip sē

nerve is _____.

4-90

In some cases of lithiasis, it may be necessary to crush calculi so they may be passed. A word to mean surgical crushing of stones, as in the bladder or ureters, is

lith/o/tripsy
lith' ō trip sē

_____.

4-91

Therapeutic ultrasound may be used to fragment stones in the kidney. This is also called

lithotripsy

_____.

ANSWER COLUMN

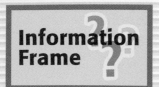

Information Frame

4-92

-iasis is a suffix used to indicate a pathological condition. -iasis may also be used when an infestation has occurred; i.e., stones, parasites, fungi.

4-93

Lith/iasis is a disease condition characterized by the presence of stones (calculi). The presence of gallstones in the gallbladder is called:

chol/e/lith/iasis
kō lē li **thi′** ə sis

_____.

4-94

Look up the following terms in your medical dictionary. What is the "organism" that causes each condition?

trichomonas
yeast (monilia)
filarial worm

trichomoniasis _____
moniliasis _____
elephantiasis _____.

4-95

Bile (gall) is secreted by the gallbladder. Chol/e/cyst is a medical name for the _____.
The combining form is **cholecyst/o**.

gallbladder

4-96

Recall that -gram refers to a picture and -graphy refers to the process of taking a picture or recording.
Build terms from the following meanings:
an x-ray of the gallbladder

_____;

chol/e/cyst/o/gram
kō′ lē sis **tō′** gram

the process of taking a gallbladder x-ray

_____;

chol/e/cyst/o/graphy
kō′ lē sis **tog′** ra fē

X-ray of a gallbladder

4-97

Gallstones can result in inflammation of the gallbladder (chol/e/cyst).
Medically, this is called _____.

chol/e/cyst/itis
kō′ lē sis **tī′** tis

ANSWER COLUMN

4-98

Cholecystitis is accompanied by pain and hyperemesis. Fatty foods aggravate these symptoms and should be avoided in cases of

cholecystitis

_____ .

4-99

When a cholelith causes cholecystitis, surgery may be needed. One surgical procedure is an incision into the gallbladder, called a

chol/e/cyst/otomy
kō′ lē sis **tot′** ə mē
chol/e/lith/otomy
kō′ lē lith **ot′** ə mē

_____ or

_____ .

4-100

Usually the presence of a gallstone calls for the excision of the gallbladder. This is a

chol/e/cyst/ectomy
kō′ lē sis **tek′** tə mē

_____ .

4-101

pepsis is the Greek word for digestion. From this you get the suffix -pepsia to use in words about _____ .

digestion

4-102

digestion

Dys/pepsia means poor _____ .
The result of food eaten too rapidly may be

dys/pepsia
dis **pep′** shə

_____ .

4-103

"Dyspepsia" is a noun. Eating under tension also may

dyspepsia

cause _____ .

ANSWER COLUMN

4-104

Do it!

"Peptic" means related to the action of digestive juices. Look up peptic ulcer in your dictionary and write the meaning here:
*_____.

4-105

bad, painful, or
  difficult

dys means *_____.

The opposite of dys is eu. eu means

well, easy, or good

*_____.

4-106

Form the word that means the opposite of:
dys/pepsia (poor or painful digestion)

eu/pepsia
yōō **pep'** sē ə

_____;

dys/pnea (difficult or painful breathing)

eu/pnea
yōōp **nē'** ə

_____.

4-107

Form the opposite of:
dys/kinesi/a (painful movement)

eu/kinesia
yōō ki **nē'** sē ə

_____;

dys/esthesi/a (painful sensation)

eu/esthesia
yōō es **thē'** sē ə

_____;

dys/phor/ia (feeling bad)

eu/phoria
yōō **fôr'** ē ə

_____.

ANSWER COLUMN

4-108

"Phagein" is the Greek word for eat. **phag/o** means

eat _____.

4-109

eats (or ingests)

A phag/o/cyte is a cell that _____
microorganisms. Phag/o/cyt/osis is the condition of

eating (or ingesting)

the cells _____ microorganisms.

4-110

-phagy and -phagia mean eating. Cyt/o/phagy (sī **tof'** ə jē) is
another way of saying

the ingestion of cells
  by phagocytes

* _____.

-phagy or -phagia

Nail biting (eating) is <u>onych o</u>_____.

4-111

Recall that -meter is a suffix for an instrument used to measure.
An instrument for measuring cells is a

cyt/o/meter
sī **tom'** ə ter

_____.

The process of measuring cells is

cyt/o/metry
sī **tom'** e trē

_____.

4-112

-stasis is a suffix meaning stopping or controlling. Stopping or
controlling cell growth is called _____.

cyt/o/stasis
sī **tos'** tə sis
cyt/o/scopy
sī **tos'** kə pē

Examination of cells is _____.

ANSWER COLUMN

---

trich/o/phagy
tri **kof'** ə jē
ortrichophagia
aer/o/phagy
air **of'** ə jē
   or acrophagia

4-113

Onych/o/phagy is nail biting. **trich/o** is the combining form for hair. A word that means hair swallowing is

_____.

Air swallowing is _aer   o_____.

---

brady/phagia
brad i **fā'** jē ə

4-114

Brady/phagia means slowness in eating. Abnormally slow swallowing is also called _____.

---

bradyphagia

4-115

From brady/phagia you find the word root **phag**, for eat. Children who play with their food while eating are exhibiting _____.

---

difficult or painful

4-116

dys- is a prefix meaning difficult or painful. "Dysphagia" means difficult swallowing. dys in dysphagia means
*_____.

---

fast or rapid

4-117

tachy- is a prefix used in words to show the opposite of slow. tachy means *_____.

---

rapid heart action

4-118

Tachy/cardia means *_____.

ANSWER COLUMN

4-119

The word for fast eating is

tachy/phagia
tak i **fā'** jē ə

_____.

Information Frame

4-120

Constipation, irritable bowel syndrome, and diverticular disease all have something in common. They are associated with slow movement of substances in the intestine, especially the colon. Although each condition is treated with different medications, all have dietary recommendations that include changes in dietary fiber intake through food choices and/or supplements and adequate amounts of water intake. Chronic lack of moisture and bulk in the feces makes it more difficult for the intestinal muscles to push the waste along. This leads to constipation, weak intestinal walls, development of pouches (diverticuli), and potential for infection.

4-121

Diverticulae are pouches that develop in the colon wall and produce diverticul/osis. Inflamed or infected diverticula (diverticulum, singular) are called

diverticul/it is
dī' ver ti kyōō **lī'** tis

_____.

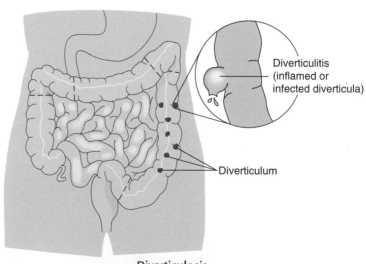

Diverticulitis
(inflamed or
infected diverticula)

Diverticulum

Diverticulosis

ANSWER COLUMN

diverticul/osis
dī' ver ti kyōō **lō'** sis

4-122

Chronic abdominal pain, cramping, and changes in bowel habits may all be symptoms of either irritable bowel syndrome or _____.

ulcers
ul' serz

4-123

Ulcers or sores in the gastrointestinal tract are another common digestive system disorder. The stomach and duodenum are the most common place for the development of _____ due to the presence of digestive juices and bacteria.

ulcers

4-124

Hemorrhage of these sores may cause a life-threatening condition requiring hospitalization. Antacids and antibiotics are often used to treat and prevent development of gastric _____.

bad

4-125

mal is a French word that means bad. mal- is also a prefix that means bad or poor. Mal/odor/ous means having a _____ odor.

poorly formed or
    poor formation

4-126

Mal/aise (mə **lāz'**) means a general feeling of illness or poor feeling. Mal/formation means *_____.

ANSWER COLUMN

4-127

Mal/nutrition means

poor nutrition

* _____.

Mal/position means

bad (abnormal)
   position or placement

* _____.

Mal/absorption means

poor absorption (as
   of nutrients)

* _____.

4-128

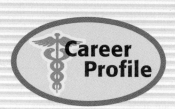

Dietetic technicians and assistants are technicians who work with dietitians to supervise the production and service of food to patients. Dietetic assistants process dietary orders, help patients select menus, and assist in food production and service.

Dietitians manage food service departments, promote health, and treat illness through nutrition education and diet planning.

NOTE: After you've "digested" and "absorbed" all the information in these frames, move on to the abbreviations, review exercises, and crossword puzzle.

ANSWER COLUMN

The following medical abbreviations correspond to the terms in Unit 4.

Abbreviation	Meaning
ac	before meals (antecibal)
BE	barium enema
BM	bowel movement
EGD	esophagogastroduodenoscopy
ERCP	endoscopic retrograde cholangiopancreatography
GB	gallbladder
GI	gastrointestinal
HAA	hepatitis-associated antigen
HBV	hepatitis B virus
NPO	nothing by mouth (nulla per os)
PO	by mouth (per os)
PC	after meals (postcibal)
UGI	upper gastrointestinal series

You have been introduced to many new terms in this unit. To make sure you know them well, work the review exercise on the following pages. Also, listen to the CD-ROM accompanying the third edition of *Medical Terminology Made Easy* and practice pronunciation.

**UNIT 4
REVIEW EXERCISE**

Part 1: Review the terms you have learned in this unit by drawing the diagonal lines between the word parts and writing the meaning of each term. Use your medical dictionary or the frames if you need help. After you have completed these tasks, say each term aloud to practice pronunciation.

1. abdominal _____

2. abdominocentesis _____

3. abdominocystic _____

4. amniocentesis _____

5. bradypepsia _____

6. cholecystectomy _____

7. cholecystogram _____

8. cholelith _____

9. cholelithiasis _____

10. colostomy _____

11. diverticulosis _____

12. duodenotomy _____

13. dysentery _____

14. dyspepsia _____

15. dysphagia _____

16. enteritis _____

17. enterorrhagia _____

18. enteroscope _____

19. esophagoduodenostomy _____

20. esophagogastric _____

21. eupepsia _____

22. gastrectomy _____

23. gastroduodenostomy _____

24. gastroenterology _____

25. gingivitis _____

26. glossitis _____

27. hemorrhage _____

UNIT 4
REVIEW EXERCISE

28. hemorrhoid _____

29. hepatomegaly _____

30. hepatopathy _____

31. hypoglossal _____

32. lithogenic _____

33. malabsorption _____

34. malnutrition _____

35. neurotripsy _____

36. pancreatolith _____

37. phagocytosis _____

38. proctologist _____

39. rectoscopy _____

40. splenectomy _____

41. splenorrhaphy _____

42. stomatalgia _____

43. stomatoscopy _____

44. sublingual _____

45. tachyphagia _____

46. ulcer _____

Part 2: Match each term with its correct meaning.

_____ 1. stomatorrhaphy

_____ 2. sublingually

_____ 3. gastrorrhagia

_____ 4. enteric

_____ 5. colostomy

_____ 6. hemorrhage

_____ 7. duodenotomy

_____ 8. proctoscopy

_____ 9. hepatitis

_____ 10. cholelithiasis

a. inflammation of the colon

b. bleeding

c. inflammation of the liver

d. stone in the pancreas

e. inflammation of the gallbladder

f. below the tongue

g. process of examining the colon

h. hemorrhage of the stomach

i. condition of stones in the gallbladder

j. fixation of a prolapsed colon

k. process of examining the rectum and anus

l. pertaining to the small intestine

m. rupture of the proctos

n. incision into the first part of the small intestine

o. suturing of the mouth

p. making a new opening in the colon

UNIT 4
REVIEW EXERCISE

Part 3: Write the medical term that means:

1. surgical puncture of the abdomen _____

2. instrument used to look into the intestine _____

3. making a new opening between the stomach and
    the first part of the small intestine _____

4. difficulty with or painful swallowing _____

5. enlargement of the spleen _____

6. pertaining to the stomach and intestine _____

7. x-ray of the gallbladder _____

8. stone in the pancreas _____

9. surgical crushing of a nerve _____

10. poor or bad nutrition _____

Part 4: Use the medical terms listed below to complete these sentences:

amniocentesis	lithotripsy	cholecystogram	peptic
dysentery	sublingually	tachyphagia	gastrorrhagia
gingivitis	colostomy	sigmoidoscopy	malnutrition

1. Bill E. Rubin had an awful pain in the upper right quadrant. His doctor ordered a
    _____ to see if he had gallstones.

2. It was outrageous that the woman's stomach was bleeding profusely. The physician wrote
    _____ on her chart. Upon endoscopy, a _____
    ulcer was seen.

3. After a trip to an underdeveloped country with poor sanitation, the couple suffered from
    amebic _____.

4. John I. Fast talked too fast, walked too fast, and, when he ate too fast too, we called it
    _____.

5. Either lack of specific nutrients (undernutrition) or too much of certain nutrients (overnutrition) in
    a person's diet may cause _____.

6. The obstetrician studied the results in the genetic testing report after the
    _____ was performed.

7. Nitroglycerin is given under the tongue, or _____.

8. Poor dental care may lead to inflammation of the gums, called _____.

UNIT 4
REVIEW EXERCISE

Part 5: Draw a line to match the abbreviation with its meaning.

1. PC   endoscopic retrograde cholangiopancreatography

2. ERCP   bowel movement

3. HAA   after meals

4. BM   nothing by mouth

5. NPO   gallbladder

6. EGD   hepatitis associated antigen

7. GB   esophagogastroduodenoscopy

UNIT 4
REVIEW EXERCISE

Part 6: Label the diagram of the digestive system. Then draw a line to the combining form matching that structure.

1. hepat/o   _____

2. gastr/o   _____

3. col/o   _____

4. esophag/o   _____

5. stomat/o   _____

6. pancreat/o   _____

7. sigmoid/o   _____

8. pharyng/o   _____

9. cholecyst/o _____

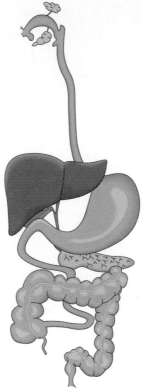

Digestive System

Unit 4 Puzzle

As a self-test work this crossword puzzle and then check your answers in Appendix F.

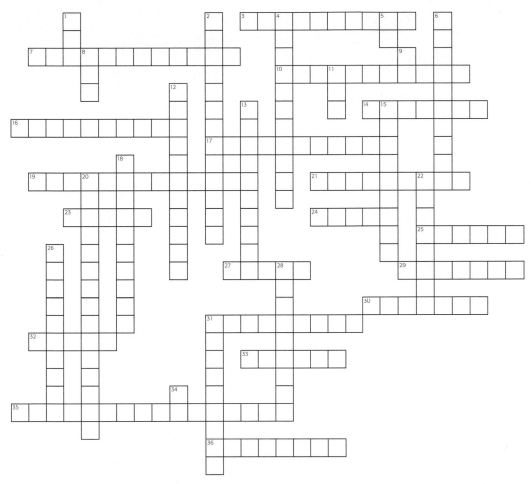

ACROSS

3. below the tongue
7. poor nutrition
10. pockets in the intestinal lining
14. pertaining to the spleen
16. inflammation of the gums
17. mouth pain
19. pancreatic stone
21. rectal herniation
23. large intestine
24. opposite of brady-
25. combining form for liver
27. sore
29. suture (suffix)
30. general feeling of ill health
31. difficult or poor digestion
32. flow or discharge (suffix)
33. hair (combining form)
35. paracentesis (synonym)
36. combining form for abdomen

DOWN

1. word root for bad
2. gallbladder inflammation
4. slow eating
5. before meals
6. below the tongue
8. nothing by mouth
9. after meals
11. esophagus, stomach, duodenum exam with a scope (abbrev.)
12. create a new opening in the stomach
13. esophagus (adj.)
15. cell that eats cells
18. bleed
20. excision of the gallbladder
22. feeling good
26. blood vessel dilation of a vein (rectal)
28. inflammation of the small intestine
31. specialist who manages diets
34. barium enema

UNIT 5
Muscles, Bones, and Joints

Study these word parts, meanings, and examples. Then proceed to the first frame.

COMBINING FORMS
acromi/o (acromion process)
arthr/o (joint)
calcane/o (heel bone)
carp/o (carpal bone)
cervic/o (cervical, neck)
chondr/o (cartilage)
clavicul/o, cleid/o (clavical)
coccyg/o (coccyx)
condyl/o (condyle)
cost/o (rib)
crani/o (skull)
dent/o (tooth)
disk/o (disk)
fibul/o (fibula)
femor/o (femur)
humer/o (humerus)
ischi/o (ischium)
kinesi/o (movement)
lamin/o (lamina)
lumb/o (lumbar spine or region)
malac/o (softening)
metacarp/o (metacarpal bone)
my/o (muscle)
odont/o (teeth)
orth/o (straight)
oste/o (bone)
pelv/i, pelv/o (pelvic)
phalang/o (phalanges)
por/o (porous)
pub/o (pubis)

radi/o (radius)
rheumat/o (rheumatism)
sacr/o (sacrum)
stern/o (sternum)
ten/o, tendon/o, tendin/o (tendon)
thorac/o (thorax)
tibi/o (tibia)
uln/o (ulna)
xiph/o (xiphoid process)

PREFIXES
de- (down from, less than)
dys- (difficulty or painful)
epi- (upon)
inter- (between)
meta- (beyond)
peri- (around, near)
supra- (above or on the topside)

SUFFIXES
-ar, al, ic (adjective endings)
-centesis (surgical puncture)
-ist (specialist)
-meter (instrument used to measure)
-metry (process of measuring)
-oid (resembling, like)
-plasia (development)
-plasty (surgical repair)
-plegia (paralysis)
-scope (instrument for looking)
-scopy (process of examination with a scope)

Word Examples

COMBINING FORMS

acromioclavicular
arthritis
calcaneodynia
metacarpals
cervicobrachial
hypochondriac
clavicular
coccygeal
epi condyle
intercostal
craniomalacia
dentoid
diskectomy
fibuloplasty
femoral
humeroscapular
ischiopubic
kinesiology
laminectomy
lumbosacral
malacotomy
metacarpophalangeal
myocardium
periodontal
orthodontist
osteoarthritis
pelvimetry
phalangitis
osteoporosis
pubic

radioulnar
rheumatoid
sacroiliac
substernal
tendonitis
thoracocentesis
tibial
ulnohumeral
xiphosternal

PREFIXES

decalcification
dysplasia
epichondral
intercostal
metatarsals
periosteum
suprapubic

SUFFIX

condylar
thoracocentesis
dentist
craniometer
craniometry
myoid
chondrodysplasia
tendonoplasty
myoplegia
arthroscope
arthroscopy

ANSWER COLUMN

5-1

PRONUNCIATION NOTE:

Now that you are learning more complex terms, it is time to suggest a way to remember some commonly mispronounced words. Begin with the suffixes -scope and -scopy. -scope is pronounced just as it looks: arthroscope (**är'** thrō skōp), endoscope (**en'** dō skōp). But -scopy is not pronounced as it looks. The "o" from the combining form blends with the suffix and is a **short** "o" sound, as in "ostrich" or "optical." The accent is also placed on this vowel–suffix blend:

arthroscopy (är **thros'** ko pē)
endoscopy (end **os'** ko pē)

Many other suffixes follow a similar pattern, for example:

-pathy	**op'** athy	-trophy	**ot'** rophy
-lysis	**ol'** ysis	-graphy	**og'** raphy
-stasis	**os'** tasis	-metry	**om'** etry
-meter	**om'** eter	-tomy	**ot'** omy
-stomy	**os'** tomy	-rrhaphy	**orr'** haphy
-logy	**ol'** ogy		

Refer back to this list as you learn these suffixes.

5-2

oste

oste/o/pathy

os tē **op'** ə thē

Oste/o/pathy means disease of the bones. From this word, form the word root for bone: _____.
Any disease of a bone is _____.

5-3

oste/itis

os tē **ī'** tis

A word meaning inflammation of bones is

_____.

ANSWER COLUMN

5-4

oste/o is the combining form for bone. -malacia is a suffix for softening. Oste/o/malacia means softening of the bones. To say that bones have lost a detectable amount of their hardness, use the noun

oste/o/malacia
os' tē ō mə **lā'** shē ə

_____.

5-5

One cause of oste/o/malacia is low intake of phosphorus and calcium. The adult equivalent of rickets characterized by soft bones is called _____.

osteomalacia

5-6

Recall that **crani/o** means skull. Build a word meaning: softening of the skull _____.

crani/o/malacia
krān' ē ō mə **lā'** shē ə

5-7

Form a word that means disease of bone:

oste/o/pathy
os' tē **op'** ə thē

_____.

5-8

A hard outgrowth on a bone may be a bone tumor, or

_____.

A cancerous tumor of the bone is

oste/oma
os' tē **ō** ma
oste/o/sarcoma
os' tē ō sar **cō'** mə

_____. **Oste/o** is used in words to mean bone.

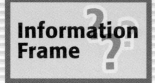

Information Frame

5-9

Falls, bumps, crashes, and disease that put stress on bones often cause cracks and breaks called fractures. Study the following table to learn about how these fractures are described, then refer to the illustration below.

FRACTURE FACTS

Complete	through the width of the bone
Incomplete	not through the width of the bone
Closed	also called simple (skin is not broken)
Open	also called compound (bone ends protrude through open skin)
Pathologic	diseased area that weakens the bone
Fracture reduction and fixation	
Closed manipulation	movement of body part to cause bone ends to align without surgery
Open manipulation	movement of body part to cause bone alignment with surgery
Internal fixation	screws or nails in bone under the skin
External fixation	screws attached to an external bar

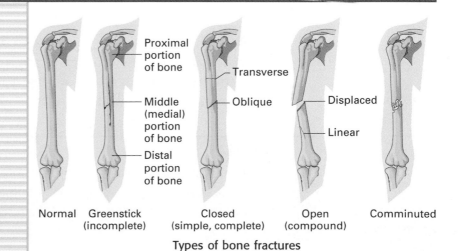

Types of bone fractures

Normal   Greenstick (incomplete)   Closed (simple, complete)   Open (compound)   Comminuted

Proximal portion of bone
Middle (medial) portion of bone
Distal portion of bone
Transverse
Oblique
Displaced
Linear

ANSWER COLUMN

5-10

de- is a prefix meaning down from or less than. Calcification is the process of adding calcium to bone structure. When calcium is removed from the bones, there is less calcium than before. This process is called

de/calcification
dē kal′ si fi **kā′** shən

_____.

5-11

Decalcification can occur from many causes. When a pregnant woman does not eat enough calcium for the growing baby, her own bones may be robbed of calcium,

decalcification

and _____ may occur.

5-12

Oste/o/por/osis is a disease condition of the bone in which there is deterioration of the bone matrix. Calcium deficiency and hormone changes associated with menopause in women with a hereditary predisposition may lead to _____.

oste/o/por/osis
os′ tē ō pə **rō′** sis

5-13

Decalcification may also occur if a person is too sedentary. Regular weight-bearing exercise, such as walking, may also help prevent

oste/o/por/osis

_____.

5-14

arthr/o is the combining form for joint. An instrument used to look at something is a scope. An instrument

arthr/o/scope
är′ thrō skōp

used to look into a joint is an _____.

ANSWER COLUMN

5-15

-scope is the suffix used to indicate the instrument used to look into body cavities, vessels, and joints. To indicate the process of using a scope, use the suffix -scopy. The process of looking into a joint with a scope is called _____.

arthr/o/scopy
är **thros'** ko pē

5-16

Arthr/o/scopy enables the physician to see into a joint area and view the injury or disease. Before surgery on a joint, the physician will perform _____ to diagnose the joint problem.

arthr/o/scopy

5-17

Spell Check

You have now learned three word parts that are often misspelled and confused because of their similarities. **Arteri/o, ather/o**, and **arthr/o** look very much alike, but their meanings are very different. Copy each below and then write an example of a word using each next to the word part for practice:

	word part	example
arteri/o	_____	_____
ather/o	_____	_____
arthr/o	_____	_____

5-18

Oste/o/arthr/o/pathy is a noun that means any disease involving bones and joints. **arthr/o** is used in words to mean _____.

joint

ANSWER COLUMN

5-19

Oste/o/arthr/o/pathy is a compound noun. Analyze it:

oste/o

_____ bone (combining form)

arthr/o

_____ joint (combining form)

pathy

_____ disease (suffix)

Now put it together:

oste/o/arthr/o/pathy

_____.

os' tē ō är **throp'** ə thē

5-20

Plastic surgery has nothing to do with plastic (the material). The word root **plast** means form or rebuild. Think of a plast/ic surgeon building a new nose or doing a face-lift. The suffix used to indicate surgical repair is

plasty

_____.

5-21

Surgical repair of a joint is

arthr/o/plasty

_____.

är' thrō plas' tē

5-22

Arthr/o/plasty may take many forms. When a joint has lost its ability to move, movement can sometimes be

arthroplasty

restored by an _____.

5-23

Orth/o/ped/ists are physician specialists in the care of bone and joint disease who perform arthroplasty while looking into a joint using an instrument called an

arthr/o/scope

_____.

är' thrō skōp

ANSWER COLUMN

5-24

Form a word that means inflammation of a joint:

arthr/itis
är **thrī'** tis

_____.

5-25

joints

oste/o/arthr/itis
os' te ō är **thrī'** tis

Rheumat/oid arthritis and oste/o/arthr/itis are both
conditions involving _____. The type
of arthritis associated with bone degeneration is

_____.

5-26

Rheumat/ism includes many different conditions that are
characterized by inflammation, degeneration, and connective
tissue changes, especially in the joints. This type of condition in
the joint is called

rheumat/oid
rōō' mə toid
arthr/itis
är **thrī'** tis

_____

_____.

5-27

rheumat/o/logist
rōō' mə **tol'** ō jist

A physician specialist who treats arthritic disorders is

a _____.

rheumat/o/logy
rōō' mə **tol'** ō jē

The study of thorough research and application of new treatments
for arthritis is _____.

5-28

You're getting to be good at this, aren't you?
Form a word that means incision into a joint:

arthr/o/tomy
är **throt'** ə mē

_____

ANSWER COLUMN

5-29

The word oste/o/chondr/itis means inflammation of bone and cartilage. The combining form for cartilage is _____.

chondr/o

5-30

Cartilage is a tough, elastic, connective tissue found in the ear, nose tip, and rib ends. The lining of joints also contains _____.

cartilage

5-31

Form a word meaning pain in or around cartilage:

_____.

    (word root)   (suffix)

chondr/algia
kon **dral'** jē ə

5-32

Chondr/ectomy means

*_____.

excision of cartilage

5-33

-plasia is a suffix for development. Using myel/o/dys/plasia as a model, build a word meaning:

defective development of cartilage

_____;

defective formation of bone and cartilage

_____.

chondr/o/dys/plasia
kon' drō dis **plā'** zhə

oste/o/chondr/o/dys/plasia
os' tē ō kon' drō dis **plā'** zhə

ANSWER COLUMN

ten/o/plasty
ten′ ō plas tē

ten/algia
ten **al′** jē ə

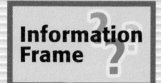

Information Frame

5-34

Ten/o is one combining form for tendon. Build a word meaning:
surgical repair of tendons

_____;

tendon pain

_____.

5-35

Tendons are made of connective tissue and attach muscle to
bone. **Ligaments** attach bone to bone, and **fascia** attaches
muscle to muscle.

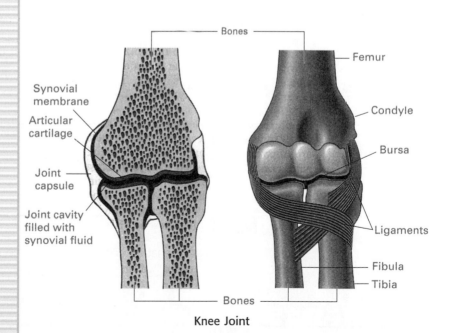

Knee Joint

ANSWER COLUMN

5-36

tendin/o and **tendon/o** are both combining forms for tendon. Use your dictionary to help build a term meaning surgical repair of the tendons

tendin/o/plasty
ten′ di nō plas′ tē

_____.

Inflammation of a tendon is:

tendon/itis
ten′ do **nī′** tis
tendin/itis
ten′ di **nī′** tis

_____

or

_____.

Note: Look at the muscle diagram on page 199 to see tendons.

5-37

Chondr/o/cost/al means pertaining to cartilage and ribs.
cost/o is used in words about the _____.

ribs

5-38

Form a word that means excision of a rib or ribs:

cost/ectomy
kos **tek′** tə mē

_____.

Note: Look at the skeletal diagram on page 190 to see the rib cage.

5-39

Chondr/o/cost/al is an adjective. This is evident because
al is the ending for an _____.

adjective

5-40

Form a word that means pertaining to the ribs:

cost/al
kos′ təl

_____.

5-41

Inter/cost/al means **between** the ribs. The prefix for
"between" is _____.

inter-

EXAMPLE: International means **between** nations.

ANSWER COLUMN

5-42

Form an adjective that means pertaining to between cartilages: _____.

inter/chondr/al
in tər **kon'** drəl

5-43

Inter/cost/al means pertaining to between the ribs.
inter- is the prefix that means _____.

between

5-44

Inter/cost/al may refer to pertaining to the muscles between the ribs. The muscles that move the ribs when breathing are the _____ muscles.

inter/cost/al
in tər **kos'** təl

5-45

dent/o is one combining form for teeth. Inter/dent/al means pertaining to between the teeth. The word root for tooth is _____.

dent

5-46

Form an adjective that means pertaining to the teeth.
_____

dent/al
den' təl

5-47

Pain in the teeth, or a toothache, is called _____.

dent/algia
den **tal'** jē ə

ANSWER COLUMN

5-48

Recall that -oid is the suffix that means like or resembling.
Form a word that means tooth-shaped, or resembling a tooth.

dent/oid
den' toid

_____

5-49

teeth
teeth

A dent/ist takes care of _____.
A dent/ifrice is used for cleaning _____.

5-50

orth is a word root taken from the Greek word "orthos," meaning
straight. **odont/o** (odonto) is another combining form for teeth.
A dentist who specializes in straightening abnormally positioned
teeth is called an

orth/odont/ist
ōr' thō **don'** tist

_____.

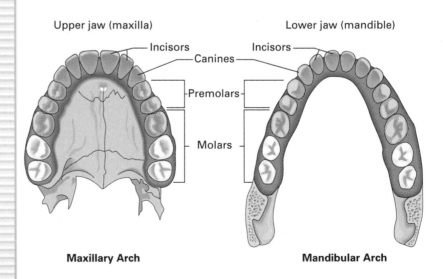

Upper jaw (maxilla)   Lower jaw (mandible)

Incisors
Canines
Premolars
Molars

Incisors

Maxillary Arch   **Mandibular Arch**

Deciduous teeth

ANSWER COLUMN

5-51

From the original Greek meaning "to straighten the child," orth/o/pedics is the specialty pertaining to the correction of deformities in the musculoskeletal system. The physician who performs surgery on the skeletal system

orth/o/ped/ist
ōr′ thō **pēd′** ist

is an _____.

5-52

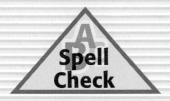

Spell Check

An alternative old Greek spelling is orthopaedics and orthopaedist. The "ae" is still pronounced like an "ē."

5-53

peri- is a prefix meaning around or near. Peri/odont/al

around or near

disease is disease * _____ the teeth.

5-54

Surgery of the gums (the tissues around the teeth) is

peri/odont/al
pair′ ē ō **don′** təl

_____ surgery.

ANSWER COLUMN

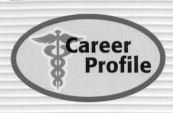

5-55

Dentistry has many branches. General dentistry performed by a **Doctor of Dental Surgery** (DDS) is dedicated to maintaining and promoting good oral health. If the dental pulp or tooth root is injured or infected, an end/odont/ist may perform the necessary treatment. A peri/odont/ist specializes in treating diseases of the tissues surrounding the teeth, such as performing a gingivectomy and an orth/odont/ist uses braces and other appliances to straighten teeth.

5-56

Name the dentist that:
straightens teeth

orth/odont/ist
or tho **don'** tist

_____;

treats disease of tissues around the teeth

peri/odont/ist
pair e o **don'** tist

_____;

treats disorders of the dental pulp and root

end/odont/ist
en do **don'** tist

_____.

5-57

lumb/o builds words about the lower back. Lumb/ar is the adjectival form. An adjective meaning pertaining to

lumb/ar
lum' bär

the lower back is _____.

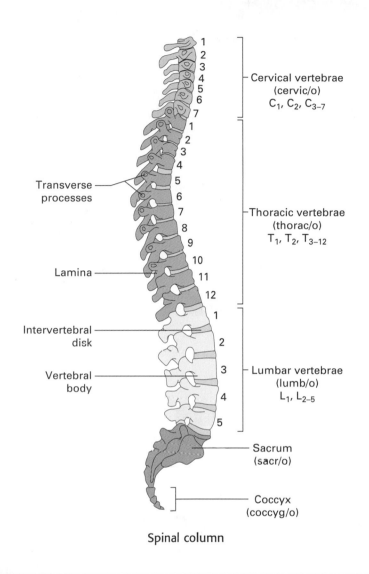

Spinal column

5-58

lumbar

There are five lumb/ar vertebrae. Low back pain is
called _____ pain.

5-59

lumbar

There is also a reflex of the lower back called the
_____ reflex.

ANSWER COLUMN

5-60

thorac/o is the combining form for chest or thorax.
Thorac/o/lumb/ar is a(n) (choose one)

adjective
pertaining to the chest
    and lower back

_____ (noun/adjective)
meaning *_____.

5-61

A word that means any chest disease is

thorac/o/pathy
thôr′ ə **kop′** ə thē

_____.

5-62

Build a term meaning pertaining to the thoracic and
lumbar vertebrae: _____.

thorac/o/lumbar
thôr′ ak ō **lum′** bar

5-63

A word that means incision of the chest is

thorac/o/tomy
thôr′ ə **kot′** ə mē

_____.

5-64

Centesis is a suffix for a surgical puncture to remove fluid from
a cavity. A word that means surgical tapping of the chest to
remove fluids is

thorac/o/centesis
thôr′ ə kō sen **tē′** sis

_____.

     (surgical puncture)

5-65

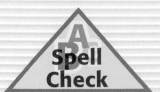

Usually, thoracocentesis is shortened to thoracentesis
(thor′ a sen **tē′** sis). Find out what form your local hospital uses.

ANSWER COLUMN

5-66

Do it!

The spinal column is divided into five regions that include the cervical, thoracic, lumbar, sacral, and coccyx, or tail, bones. Look at the diagram of the spinal column and count how many vertebrae (back bones) are in each region.

7
12
5
5 fused
3

Cervical _____

Thoracic _____

Lumbar _____

Sacral _____

Coccyx _____

5-67

The terms "thoracic" and "lumbar" are also used to describe regions of the abdomen. The thorax is the chest and the right and left lumbar regions are at the waist. Refer to the diagram of the regions in Unit 9 on page 332.

5-68

heart cavity
   (pericardium)
abdomen
a surgical puncture
   of the lung cavity
   to remove fluid

A cardi/o/centesis is a surgical puncture of the

* _____.

An abdomin/o/centesis is the surgical puncture of the

_____.

A pleurocentesis is ** _____.

5-69

Information
Frame

supra- is a prefix that means above, over, or on the top side.

5-70

supra-

Supra/lumb/ar means above the lumbar region. A prefix that means above is _____.

ANSWER COLUMN

5-71

above the lumbar region or
above the lower back

Supra/lumb/ar means *_____

_____.

5-72

above the ribs

Supra/cost/al means *_____

_____.

5-73

Supra/crani/al refers to the surface of the head

on top of

*_____ the skull.

5-74

The pub/is is a bone of the pelvis. Pub/is is a (choose

noun

one) _____ (noun/adjective).

5-75

From **pub/o** form

pubis
pubic

a noun _____;
an adjective _____.

5-76

pubes
pyoō′ bēz

Locate the pubis. The plural of pubis is _____.
of pubis is _____.

5-77

Recall that **rect/o** means rectum. Using **pub/o** and **rect/o**, build a
word meaning: pertaining to the pubis and the

pub/o/rect/al
pyoō bō **rek′** təl

rectum: _____.

ANSWER COLUMN

5-78

pubis

pub/o in a word refers to the _____.
(You did that one by yourself.)

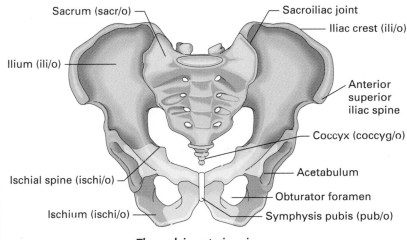

Sacrum (sacr/o)

Sacroiliac joint

Iliac crest (ili/o)

Ilium (ili/o)

Anterior
superior
iliac spine

Coccyx (coccyg/o)

Acetabulum

Ischial spine (ischi/o)

Obturator foramen

Ischium (ischi/o)

Symphysis pubis (pub/o)

The pelvis anterior view

5-79

pub/is
pyoo′ bis

The pub/ic bone is also called the _____.

5-80

pubis

Supra/pub/ic means above the pubis. **Pub/o** is used in words about
the _____.

5-81

supra/pub/ic
soo prə **pyoo′** bik

The suprapubic region is above the arch of the pub/is. When the
bladder is incised above the pubis, an incision is made in the
_____ region.

ANSWER COLUMN

pelv/is **pel'** vis	**5-82** The pelv/is is formed by the pelv/ic bones, including the ilium, ischium and pubis. **Pelv/i** refers to the _____ (noun).
pelv/i/metry pel **vim'** ə trē	**5-83** Pelv/i/metry is done during pregnancy to find the measurements of the pelvis. To find a woman's pelvic size, the physician does _____.
pelvimetry	**5-84** A physician may determine whether or not a woman may have trouble during labor by doing _____.
pelv/i/meter pel **vim'** ə tər	**5-85** Look in the dictionary for a word that names the device used for pelvimetry. It is a _____.
supra/pelv/ic soo prə **pel'** vik	**5-86** The adjective meaning **above** the pelvis is _____.
instrument instrument pelvis	**5-87** Recall that -meter is an instrument to measure. A speed/o/meter is an _____ to measure speed. A pelv/i/meter is an _____ to measure the _____.

ANSWER COLUMN

5-88

measures (counts),
  cells

measures, head

thorac/o/meter

thôr′ ə **kom′** ə tər

cardi/o/meter

kär dē **om′** ə tər

A cyt/o/meter _____ the
_____. A cephal/o/meter
_____ the _____.

A _____ measures the chest.

A _____ measures the heart.

5-89

ischia

is′ kē ə

Refer to the illustration on page 187. Locate the ischium of the
pelvis. The plural of ischium is _____.

5-90

ischi

From "ischium" and "ischia," derive a word root that refers to the
part of the hip bone on which the body rests when sitting.
The word root is _____.

5-91

ischi/o

Look up words that begin with **ischi**. The combining form used in
words to refer to the ischium is _____.

5-92

ischi/o/rect/al

is′ kē ō **rek′** təl

ischi/o/pub/ic

is′ kē ō **pyoō′** bik

In your dictionary, find a word meaning: pertaining to ischium and
rectum

_____;

pertaining to the ischium and pubis

_____.

ANSWER COLUMN

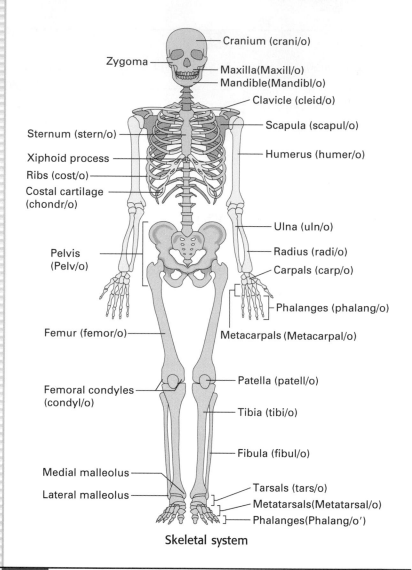

Cranium (crani/o)

Zygoma

Maxilla(Maxill/o)

Mandible(Mandibl/o)

Clavicle (cleid/o)

Scapula (scapul/o)

Sternum (stern/o)

Humerus (humer/o)

Xiphoid process

Ribs (cost/o)

Costal cartilage (chondr/o)

Ulna (uln/o)

Radius (radi/o)

Pelvis (Pelv/o)

Carpals (carp/o)

Phalanges (phalang/o)

Femur (femor/o)

Metacarpals (Metacarpal/o)

Patella (patell/o)

Femoral condyles (condyl/o)

Tibia (tibi/o)

Fibula (fibul/o)

Medial malleolus

Lateral malleolus

Tarsals (tars/o)

Metatarsals(Metatarsal/o)

Phalanges(Phalang/o')

Skeletal system

5-93

Close your dictionary. Build a word meaning:
pertaining to the ischium

ischi/al
is' kē əl

_____ ;

herniation through the sciatic notch in the ischium

ischi/o/cele
is' kē ō sēl

_____ ;

pertaining to ischium and pubis

ischi/o/pubic
is' kē ō **pyoo'** bik

_____ .

ANSWER COLUMN

ischium
is' kē əm

5-94

ischi/o in a word refers to the part of the hip bone called the _____.

Information Frame

5-95

Combining Form	Noun	Adjective
cervic/o	neck, cervical vertebrae	cervical
thorac/o	thorax	thoracic
ili/o	ilium	iliac
sacr/o	sacrum	sacral
coccyg/o	coccyx	coccygeal
lumb/o	lumbus	lumbar

Refer to the diagram of the spine on page 183.

cervical
cervical

5-96

A device used to immobilize the neck, such as after a whiplash injury, is a _____ collar.
The vertebrae of the neck are the _____ vertebrae.

sacr/o/iliac
sāk rō **il'** ē ak   or
ili/o/sacr/al
il' ē ō **sāk'** rəl

5-97

The joint between the sacrum and the ilium is the _____ joint.

ANSWER COLUMN

5-98

Build a term meaning:
pertaining to the sacrum and the sciatic nerve

sacr/o/sciatic
sāk′ rō sī **a**′ tik

_____;

removal of the coccyx

coccyg/ectomy
kok′ si **jek**′ tə mē

_____.

5-99

disk is the word root indicating intervertebral disk. Look at the diagram on page 183 of the spinal column to locate the lamina and intervertebral disk. A myel/o/gram (spinal x-ray) is used to diagnose disk herniation. Removal of a herniated disk is

disk/ectomy
dis **kek**′ tə mē

called a _____.

lamin/ectomy
lam i **nek**′ tə mē

Removal of the lamina is called
lamin_____.

5-100

Do it!

The bones of the arm and hand include the humerus, ulna, radius, carpals, metacarpals, and phalanges. Look at the diagram of the skeleton and locate each of these bones. Notice the combining forms that are also labeled for you. Write the names of the bones on sticky labels and attach them to your body in the appropriate places to remember the locations and names.

5-101

humer/o

Look at **Frame 5–100**. Can it start you looking for the combining form for the upper arm bone? Try. It is _____

5-102

humerus

humer/o is used in words to refer to the bone of the upper arm, which is named the _____.

ANSWER COLUMN

5-103

Find three words in your dictionary that begin
with humer or humer/o. They are:

(pick three of four)
humeral
humeroradial
humeroscapular
humeroulnar

_____;
_____;
_____.

5-104

It could get to be a
   never-ending thing,
   couldn't it?

Could **Frame 5–103** start you building other combining
forms? Well, it isn't necessary, but you may if you like.

5-105

The radius **(radi/o)** and ulna **(uln/o)** are located in the forearm.
If both are fractured it would be described as a

radi/o/ulnar
rā dē **ō ul'** när

_____ fracture.

(Abbreviation: FxBB—fracture of both bones)

5-106

Locate the carpal bones. The plural of carpus is

carpi
kär' pē
or carpals
kär palz

_____.

5-107

From carpus and carpi, derive a word root that refers to
the wrist. It is _____.

carp

ANSWER COLUMN

5-108

Carpal tunnel syndrome is an occupational hazard to court reporters and others who do a lot of typing. The adjectival form for carpus is _____.

carp/al
kär' pəl

5-109

Look at the words in your medical dictionary that begin with **carp**. The combining form used in words about the wrist is _____.

carp/o

5-110

Close your dictionary. Build a word meaning:
pertaining to the wrist (adjective)
_____;

carp/al
kär' pəl

pertaining to the wrist and metacarpals (adjective)
_____;

carp/o/metacarpal
kär' pō **met'** ə kär pəl

excision of all or part of the wrist (noun)
_____.

carp/ectomy
kär **pek'** tə mē

5-111

meta means beyond. The bones in the hand "beyond" the carpals are called the _____.

meta/carpals
met ə **kär'** pəlz

5-112

Locate the phalanges. They are the *_____
_____.

bones of the fingers
  and/or toes

ANSWER COLUMN

5-113

The word root for "phalanges" is

phalang   _____.

5-114

Build a word meaning:
inflammation of phalanges

phalang/itis
fal an **jī′** tis   _____;

    excision of a phalanx (singular)

phalang/ectomy
fal an **jek′** tə mē   _____.

5-115

Congratulations!   You are now finding your own combining forms. Feels good, doesn't it? Let's do some more.

5-116

Locate the acromion. It is a projection of the

scapula   _____. Refer to the skeleton on page 190.

5-117

The combining form for the acromion process is

acromi/o   _____.

5-118

Now let's see how skilled you are at finding your own word roots and endings. Build a term that means:
pertaining to the acromion

_____;

acromi/al
a **krō'** mē əl

pertaining to the acromion and humerus

_____;

acromi/o/humer/al
a krō' mē ō **hyōō'** mər əl

pertaining to the acromion and the scapula

_____ scapular .

acromi/o/scapul/ar
a krō' mē ō **ska'** pyōō lar

5-119

The bones of the leg include the femur (femor/o), tibia (tibi/o), and fibula (fibul/o). Build a word meaning pertaining to the:
femur and tibia

_____ al;

femor/o/tibi/al
fem' or ō **tib'** ē əl

tibia and fibula

_____ ar;

tibi/o/fibul/ar
tib' ē ō **fib'** yōō lar

fibula and calcaneus

_____ al.

fibul/o/calcane/al
fib' yōō lō kal **kān'** ē əl

5-120

Locate the calcaneus. The plural of calcaneus is

_____. From calcaneus and

calcanei
kal **kā'** nē ī

calcaneal, derive the word root for the heel:

calcane

_____.

5-121

In your medical dictionary, look at the words beginning with calcane. Derive the combining form used in words

calcane/o

that refer to the heel: _____.

ANSWER COLUMN

5-122

Close your dictionary. Now build a word meaning: pertaining to the heel _____.

calcane/al
kal **kā'** nē əl

5-123

With your dictionary open, find a word meaning: pertaining to the sternum and pericardium

_____;

stern/o/peri/cardi/al
ster' nō per i **kard'** ē əl

pertaining to the sternum and ribs

_____.

stern/o/cost/al
ster' nō **kos'** təl

5-124

Close the dictionary. Build a word meaning:
pertaining to the sternum

_____;

stern/al
ster' nəl

pain in the sternum

_____.

stern/algia
stern **al'** jē ə

5-125

stern/o in a word makes you think of the
_____, which is the

sternum
breastbone
_____.

5-126

The **xiphoid** (swordlike) process is the projection at the inferior end of the sternum. **xiph/o** is the combining form. A word meaning pertaining to the xiphoid process and the ribs is

xiph/o/cost/al
zī' fō **kos'** təl
_____.

ANSWER COLUMN

5-127

Refer back to the drawing of the skeleton on page 190. Locate a condyle. A condyle is a rounded process that occurs on many bones. The word root for condyle is _____.

condyl

5-128

Build a word meaning:
excision of a condyle

condyl/ectomy
kon′ di **lek′** tə mē

_____;

resembling a condyle

condyl/oid
kon′ di loid

_____;

above a condyle

epi/condyle
ep i **kon′** dīl

_epi_____.

5-129

Condyl/ar is an adjective meaning pertaining to a
_____.

condyle
kon′ dīl

5-130

"Myocarditis" means inflammation of the heart muscle.
My/o is used in words referring to the

muscles

_____.

ANSWER COLUMN

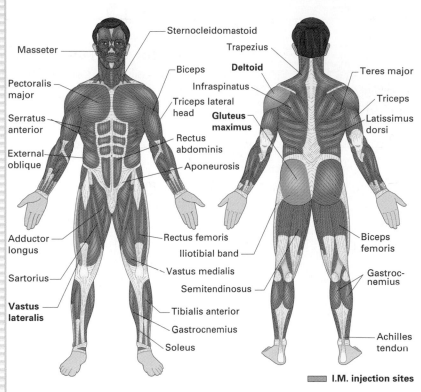

I.M. injection sites

Anterior and Posterior Views of the Muscles

5-131

Using the words "myogram," "myograph," and "myography," fill in the blanks.

myogram

myograph

myography

_____ the chart

_____ the instrument

_____ the process

5-132

muscles

my/asthenia gravis is a condition of the _____.

ANSWER COLUMN

5-133

Using **my/o**, **fibr/o**, and **oma**, build a term meaning a fibrous muscle tumor (typically found in the uterus):

my/o/fibr/oma
mī ō fīb **rō'** mə

_____, which is also called lieomyoma.

5-134

Build a word meaning:
resembling muscle

my/oid
mī' oid

_____;

muscle and fat tumor

my/o/lip/oma
mī' ō lip **ō'** mə

_____;

muscle disease

my/o/pathy
mī **op'** ath ē

_____.

5-135

For your own interest, count how many words you know beginning with **my/o**. Write the number here.

over 60

** _____

5-136

When you see **my/o**, you will think of

muscles

_____.

ANSWER COLUMN

5-137

kinesi/o is used in words to mean movement or motion.
Brady/kinesia means

slowness of
   movement

* _____

_____ .

5-138

Kinesi/algia means

pain on movement
or
movement pain

* _____

_____ .

5-139

Kinesi/algia occurs when you have to move any sore or injured part
of the body. Moving a broken arm causes

kinesi/algia
ki′ nē sē **al′** jē ə

_____ .

5-140

An exercise physiologist studies the science of how the
body moves, called _____ .

kinesi/o/logy
ki nēs ē **ol′** ə jē

5-141

Recall that brady- is the prefix for slow. Slowness of
movement is called _____ .

brady/kinesia
brad′ i kin **ēs′** ē ə

ANSWER COLUMN

The following medical abbreviations correspond to the terms in Unit 5.

Abbreviation	Meaning
C1, C2, C3 ... C7	cervical vertebrae, first, second, and so on
Ca (Ca^{++} ion)	calcium
CPD	cephalo pelvic disproportion
CXR	chest x-ray
DDS	doctor of dental surgery
DO	doctor of osteopathy
Dx	diagnosis
Fx	fracture
FxBB	fracture of both bones
L1, L2, ... L5	lumbar vertebrae, first, second, and so on
OA	osteoarthritis
OREF	open reduction external fixation
ORIF	open reduction internal fixation
Orth, ortho	orthopedist
RA	rheumatoid arthritis
T1, T2, T3, ... T12	thoracic vertebrae, first, second, and so on

You have been introduced to many new terms in this unit. To make sure you know them well, work the review exercises on the following pages. Also, listen to the CD-ROM accompanying the third edition of *Medical Terminology Made Easy* and practice pronunciation.

UNIT 5
REVIEW EXERCISE

Part 1: Review the terms you have learned in this unit by drawing the diagonal lines between the word parts and then writing the meaning of each term. Use your medical dictionary or the frames if you need help. After you have completed these tasks, say each term aloud to practice pronunciation.

1. acromioclavicular   _____

2. arthritis   _____

3. arthroplasty   _____

4. arthroscope   _____

5. arthrotomy   _____

6. bradykinesia   _____

7. calcaneal   _____

8. carpectomy   _____

9. chondralgia   _____

10. chondrodysplasia   _____

11. costectomy   _____

12. decalcification   _____

13. dental   _____

14. dentalgia   _____

15. diskectomy   _____

16. endodontist   _____

17. epicondyle   _____

18. humeroscapular   _____

19. interchondral   _____

20. intercostal   _____

21. ischiocele   _____

22. ischiorectal   _____

23. kinesiology   _____

24. metacarpals   _____

25. myofibroma   _____

26. myography   _____

UNIT 5
REVIEW EXERCISE

27. orthodontist _____

28. orthopedist _____

29. osteitis _____

30. osteoarthritis _____

31. osteoarthropathy _____

32. osteoma _____

33. osteomalacia _____

34. osteopathy _____

35. osteoporosis _____

36. pelvimetry _____

37. periodontal _____

38. phalangitis _____

38. puborectal _____

40. radioulnar _____

41. rheumatology _____

42. sacroiliac _____

43. sternopericardial _____

44. supralumbar _____

45. tendinitis _____

46. tendonoplasty _____

47. thoracocentesis _____

48. thoracolumbar _____

49. tibiofibular _____

50. xiphocostal _____

UNIT 5
REVIEW EXERCISE

Part 2: Draw a line to match the abbreviation with its meaning.

1. Ca^{++} fracture

2. CPD   osteoarthritis

3. C_2 orthopedist

4. OA   cephalopelvic disproportion

5. DO   dentist

6. Fx   second cervical vertebra

7. DDS   calcium ion

8. ORTH   doctor of osteopathy

Part 3: Match each term with its correct meaning.

_____ 1. osteopathy   a.   resembling a sword; a bony process

_____ 2. arthroscopy   b.   instrument to measure muscle function

_____ 3. tendonoplasty   c.   between the ribs

_____ 4. chondrocostal   d.   procedure that uses an instrument to look into a joint

_____ 5. decalcification   e.   above the thorax

_____ 6. thoracolumbar   f.   any disease of the bone

_____ 7. suprapubic   g.   pertaining to cartilage and rib

_____ 8. condylar   h.   surgical repair of a tendon

_____ 9. xiphoid   i.   inflammation of a tendon

_____10. myogram   j.   resembling a xiphius

                             k.   pertaining to the thorax and lumbar spine

                             l.   taking calcium away from the bone

                             m.   above the pubic bone

                             n.   a picture of muscle function

                             o.   pertaining to a rounded, bony process

UNIT 5
REVIEW EXERCISE

Part 4: Write the medical term that means:

1. pertaining to the acromion process and the collar bone _____

2. upon the rounded part of a bone_____

3. pertaining to the sacrum and the ilium _____

4. bones in the hand beyond the wrist_____

5. muscle and fibrous tumor _____

6. surgical puncture of the chest to remove fluid _____

7. combining form for the upper arm bone_____

8. the study of movement _____

9. porous condition of the bone _____

10. dental specialist in straightening teeth _____

Part 5: Use the medical terms listed below to complete these sentences:

osteoporosis	FxBB	radioulnar	diskectomy	lumbar
chondrodysplasia	arthroscope	arthritis	xiphoid	laminectomy
ischium	intercostal	radioulnar	tendonitis	phalanx
carpal	pelvimetry			

1. Bonny Skeleton pointed the first _____ of her right hand at her skeleton teenager and said, "Are you going to sit on your _____ all day playing computer games?"

2. The tennis player complained of pain around the forearm and elbow area and knew that his _____ must have returned.

3. To confirm the diagnosis of joint inflammation called degenerative _____, the orthopedist used the _____ to examine the patient's knee joint.

4. The obstetrician performed _____ to determine pelvic size in order to be sure there would not be cephalopelvic disproportion complicating delivery of the fetus.

5. After typing medical transcriptions all day, Mr. Dick Tater's wrists were sore and his fingers were going numb. These were symptoms of his chronic fight with _____ tunnel syndrome.

6. The neurosurgeon consulted with the orthopedist to determine whether or not the patient should have a _____ or _____ to repair the herniated disk in his neck.

7. Raymond Racer was not wearing wrist guards while skateboarding and fell, breaking both bones (Abbrev. _____) in his forearm. Dx: _____ fracture.

UNIT 5
REVIEW EXERCISE

Part 6: Label the structures of the skeleton. Then draw a line to the combining form that matches that structure.

1. xiph/o _____

2. condyl/o _____

3. femor/o _____

4. cleid/o _____

5. phlang/o _____

6. carp/o _____

7. radi/o _____

8. humer/o _____

9. cost/o _____

10. scapul/o _____

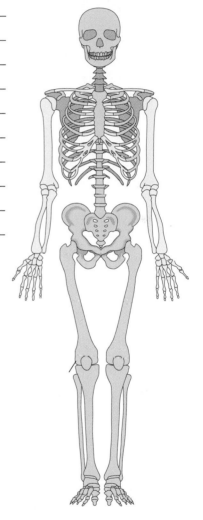

Unit 5 Puzzle

As a self-test work the crossword puzzle and then check your answers in Appendix F.

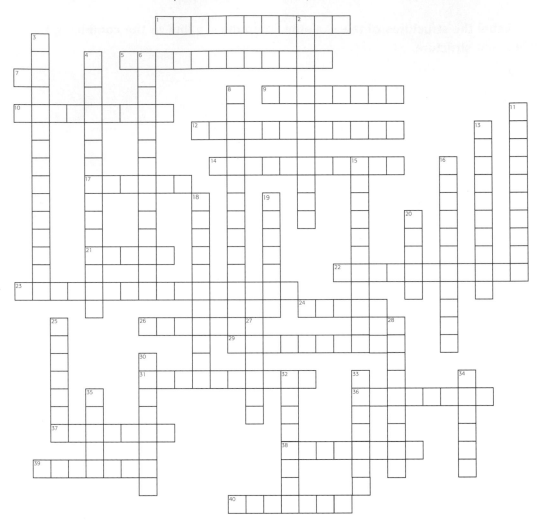

ACROSS

1. study of movement
5. joint repair
7. osteopathic physician (abbrev.)
9. pertaining to the chest
10. heel bone
12. dentist who straightens teeth
14. using an arthroscope
17. combining form for femur
21. shin bone
22. bones in the foot
23. disease of bones and joints
24. anterior of the pelvis
26. longest bone in the body
29. measurement of the pelvis
31. upon a rounded bony process
36. bony process at the shoulder
37. bony process at the end of the sternum
38. any disease of muscle
39. suffix for softening
40. resembling a tooth

DOWN

2. porous condition of a bone
3. surgical puncture to remove fluid from the chest
4. loss of calcium
6. physician specializing in arthritic disorders
8. between cartilage
11. inflammation of the tendon
13. pertaining to both bones of the forearm
15. physician specializing in bone and joint disorders
16. overdevelopment in size
18. pertaining to the ischium and pubis
19. synonym for hypotrophy
20. combining form for rib
25. singular of phalanges
27. connects muscle to bone
28. process of making an image of muscle function
30. pertaining to the neck
32. connects bone to bone
33. wrist bones
34. tail bone
35. prefix for above

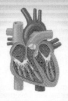 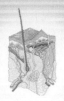

UNIT 6
Male Reproductive and Urinary Systems

Study these word parts, meanings, and examples. Then proceed to the first frame.

COMBINING FORMS

albumin/o (protein)
balan/o (glans penis)
crypt/o (hidden)
cyst/o (bladder)
glyc/o (sugar)
hem/o, hemat/o (blood)
hydr/o (water)
ket/o (ketones)
nephr/o (kidney, nephron)
noct/i, nyct/o (night)
orchid/o, orchi/o, orch/o (testis)
prostat/o (prostate)
pyel/o (renal pelvis)
ren/o (kidney)
sperm/o (sperm)
spermat/o (sperm)
ur/o (urine, urinary)
ureter/o (ureter)
urethr/o (urethra)
vas/o (vessel, vas deferens)

PREFIXES

de- (down from, less than normal)
ex- (out of)
in- (not, in)
poly- (too much, too many)

SUFFIXES

-cide (kill)
-cyst (bladder, sac)
-dynia (pain)
-ism (condition, theory)
-philia (attraction)
-phobia (fear)
-ptosis (prolapse)
-rrhagia (hemorrhage)
-rrhaphy (suture)
-rrhea (flow, discharge)
-scopy (process of looking using a scope)
-stomy (making a new opening)
-uria (in the urine)

Word Examples

COMBINING FORMS

albuminuria
balanoplasty
cryptorchidism
cystoscopy
glycosuria
hemorrhage
hydrophobia
ketosis
nephropexy
nyctalopia
orchidocele
prostatorrhea
pyelonephritis
renogram
spermolysis
spermatoid
urology
ureterolith
urethritis
vasotripsy

PREFIXES

dehydration
expiration
incontinence
polycystic

SUFFIXES

spermicide
cystorrhagia
orchidodynia
cryptorchidism
hydrophilia
hematophobia
nephroptosis
ureterorrhagia
cystorrhaphy
balanorrhea
urethroscopy
urostomy
ketouria

ANSWER COLUMN

6-1

"Sperma" is the Greek word meaning seed. **spermat/o** and **sperm/o** are two combining forms for spermatozoa or male germ cells (sperm). -genesis means growth or formation. Spermat/o/genesis means

formation of sperm

or

formation of male
   germ cells

*_____

_____.

6-2

Give a word meaning:
the destruction of spermatozoa

sperm/o/lysis
sper **mol'** i sis   or
spermat/o/lysis
sper mə **tol'** i sis
spermat/o/blast
sper **mat'** ō blast   or
sperm/o/blast
sper' mō blast

_____;

an embryonic male cell

_____ blast ____.

6-3

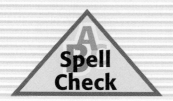

Spell
Check

The singular form is "spermatozoon." The plural form is "spermatozoa." The singular form is "sperm" and the plural form is "sperm."

ANSWER COLUMN

6-4

A bladder or sac containing sperm is a

_____.

spermat/o/cyst
sper **mat'** ō sist

A word for resembling sperm is

_____.

spermat/oid
sper' mə toid

A word for disease of the sperm is

_____.

spermat/o/pathy
sper mə **top'** ə thē

6-5

-cide is a suffix meaning to kill or destroy.
An agent used to kill sperm is a

_____.

sperm/i/cide
sper' mi sīd

ANSWER COLUMN

spermicide

6-6

Use of a condom and spermicide together is an effective birth control method. A gel or cream used to kill sperm is called a _____.

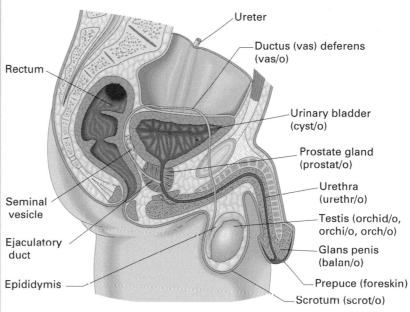

Male Reproductive System

6-7

Look up orchid/o, orchi/o, and orch/o, to discover how each is used. **orchid/o**, **orchi/o**, and **orch/o** are all combining forms for testicle. Orchid/ectomy, orchi/ectomy, and orch/ectomy all mean

excision of the
testicle

* _____

_____.

ANSWER COLUMN

6-8

Build three terms that mean pain in the testes:

orchi/algia
ôr′ kē **al′** jē a
_____;
orchid/algia
ôr′ kid **al′** jē a
_____;
orchi/o/dynia
ôr′ kē ō **din′** ē a
_____.

6-9

The adjectival form for testicle is **testicular**.
A person with orchidalgia is experiencing

testicul/ar
tes **tik′** yōo lar
_____ pain.

6-10

Testicular cancer is a serious condition that frequently afflicts
males between the ages of 18 and 35. Testicular self-exam (TSE)
and physician examination of the scrotum is recommended for
testicular
early detection of _____ cancer.

6-11

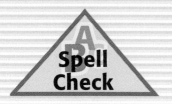

Look at the terms below. They all refer to the testes.

testis   singular noun
testes   plural noun
testicle   singular noun
testicles   plural noun
testicular   adjectival form

ANSWER COLUMN

6-12

Around the time of birth, the testicles normally descend from the abdominal cavity into the scrotum. Sometimes this fails to happen (crypt/orchid/ism). Surgical repair may be indicated. The operation is called an _____.

orchid/o/plasty
ôr′ kid ō plas′ tē

6-13

Build a word meaning:
herniation of a testicle

_____;

orchid/o/cele
ôr′ ki dō sēl

incision into a testicle

_____.

orchid/o/tomy
ôr′ kid **ot′** ə mē

6-14

Crypt/orchid/ism means undescended testicle. **crypt** means hidden. When a testicle is hidden in the abdominal cavity, the condition is known as _____.

crypt/orchid/ism
kript **ôr′** kid izm

6-15

A crypt/ic remark is one with a hidden meaning. A crypt/ic belief is one whose meaning is _____.

hidden

6-16

prostat/o is used for words relating to the prostate gland. Prostat/ic is the adjectival form, as in the condition of benign prostatic hyperplasia or prostatic hypertrophy (BPH). Build a term meaning inflammation of the prostate gland: _____.

prostat/itis
pros′ tā **tī′** tis

ANSWER COLUMN

---

prostat/o/rrhea
pros' tā tō **rē'** ə

6-17

Recall the suffix -rrhea. An abnormal flow or discharge from the prostate gland is called

_____.

---

prostat/algia
pros' tā **tal'** jē ə

6-18

Prostatic pain is called _____.

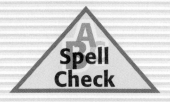

6-19

Watch the pronunciation and the spelling of prostate. It is **pros'** tāt **not pros'** trāt. Notice the spelling, too.

---

balan/o/plasty
bal' ə nō plas' tē

6-20

balan/o is the combining form for glans penis. Balanitis is inflammation of the glans penis. Surgical repair of the glans penis is called _____.

---

pen/itis
pēn **ī'** tis
pen/o/scrotal
pēn ō **skrō'** təl

6-21

pen/o is the combining form for "penis." Pen/ile is the adjective form. Inflammation of the penis is

_____.

Build a word meaning pertaining to the penis and scrotum:_____ scrotal____.

ANSWER COLUMN

to cut around
(actually a surgical
procedure for
removing the foreskin
of the penis)

6-22

From the word parts you have already learned, think of the meaning
for the following term and write it below:
circum/cision (**sûr'** kum si' shun) *_____
_____.

6-23

Vas is a word meaning vessel. **Vas/o** is another combining
form for vessel. Vas/o/dilatation means enlarging the
diameter of a _____.

vessel
ve' səl

Spell
Check

6-24

"Dilatation" and "dilation" are synonyms but spelled and pronounced
quite differently: dilatation (dil ə **tā'** shun) and dilation (**dī'** lā shun).
Also notice that dilate is pronounced **di** lat **not** dī a lāt.

decreasing the size
of the diameter
of a vessel

6-25

Vas/o/constriction is the opposite of vas/o/dilatation.
Vas/o/constriction means *_____
_____.

vessel

6-26

Vas/o/motor is an adjective that refers to nerves that control the
tone of the blood _____ walls.

ANSWER COLUMN

6-27

Using **vas/o,** build a word meaning:
pertaining to a vessel

vas/al
va′ səl, **vā′** zəl

_____;

spasm of a vessel

vas/o/spasm
vas′ ō spazm,
vā′ zō spazm

_____;

crushing of a vessel

vas/o/tripsy
vas′ ō trip sē,
vā′ zō trip sē

_____.

(with forceps to stop hemorrhage)

6-28

Look at the words used in your dictionary beginning with vas or
vas/o. Vas/o is used in words about

vessels
vas deferens
vas **def′** er enz

_____ or *_____.

6-29

Build a word meaning:
incision into the vas deferens

vas/o/tomy
vas **ot′** ə mē

_____;

suture of the vas deferens

vas/o/rrhaphy
vas **ôr′** ə fē

_____;

making a new opening into the vas deferens

vas/o/stomy
vas **os′** tə mē

_____;

removal of a segment of the vas deferens

vas/ectomy
vas **ek′** tə mē

_____.

ANSWER COLUMN

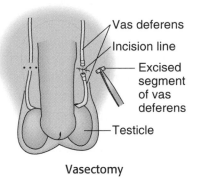

Vasectomy

Information Frame ???

6-30

ur means urine or urination. ia means condition. -uria is a suffix meaning a condition of urine or urination. Conditions involving urination include:

Word	Combining Form	Suffix to Use when Needed
urine	ur/o	-lith (stone)
kidney	nephr/o	-rrhaphy
	ren/o	(suturing or stitching)
renal pelvis	pyel/o	-rrhagia
ureter	ureter/o	(hemorrhage or "bursting forth" of blood)
bladder	cyst/o	-uria
urethra	urethr/o	(urine, urination)

6-31

Urology is the study of the **ur**inary tract. The **ur**inary tract is responsible for forming **ur**ine from waste materials in the blood and for eliminating **ur**ine from the body. What would you guess to be the word root for **ur**ine?

_____.

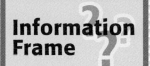

ur

ANSWER COLUMN

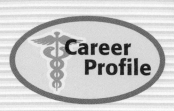

Career Profile

6-32

The physician specialist who treats male reproductive system disorders and the urinary system of both males and females is a ur/ologist (yōor **ol'** ō jist).

A urologist that specializes in treatment of kidney disorders is a nephrologist (nef **rol'** ō jist).

6-33

Build a word meaning:
pertaining to urinary tract and genitals
_____ genital;

ur/o/genital
yōor ō **jen'** i təl

any disease of the urinary tract
_____.

ur/o/pathy
yōor **op'** ə thē

6-34

nephr/o is used in words to refer to the kidney.
A word that means inflammation of the kidney is
_____.

nephr/itis
nef **rī'** tis

6-35

inflammation of
 a kidney

Nephr/itis means *_____.
Build a word meaning:
destruction of kidney tissue
_____.

nephr/o/lysis
nef **rol'** ə sis

ANSWER COLUMN

6-36

Build a word meaning:
stone in the kidney

nephr/o/lith
nef′ rō lith

_____;

softening of kidney tissue

nephr/o/malacia
nef′ rō mə **lā′** sē a

_____;

enlargement of the kidney

nephr/o/megaly
nef′ rō **meg′** ə lē

_____.

6-37

-ptosis refers to an organ that has dropped out of its normal location (prolapsed). orchid/o/ptosis is prolapse of the testicle. A prolapsed kidney is _____.

nephr/o/ptosis
nef′ rop **tō′** sis

6-38

The renal pelvis is formed at the juncture of the calyces. **pyel/o** refers to the *_____.

renal pelvis

6-39

Using what you need from the combining form for renal pelvis, form words meaning:
inflammation of the renal pelvis

pyel/itis
pī ə **lī′** tis

_____;

surgical repair of the renal pelvis

pyel/o/plasty
pī′ ə lō plas′ tē

_____.

ANSWER COLUMN

6-40

condition of renal
  pelvis and kidney
pyel/o/nephr/itis
pī′ ə lō ne **frī′** tis

Pyel/o/nephr/osis means *_____.
Form a word that means inflammation of the renal pelvis and kidney:
_____.

6-41

Using the table on page 219, give the meaning of:

stone or calculus
  in the ureter

ureter/o/lith *_____.
Then form a word that means:
hemorrhage of the ureter

ureter/o/rrhagia
yōō **rē′** ter ō **rā′** jē ə

_____;

suturing of the ureter

ureter/o/rrhaphy
yōō rē ter **ôr′** ə fē

_____;

prolapse of a ureter

ureter/o/ptosis
yōō rē′ ter op **tō′** sis

_____.

6-42

suturing or stitching
  of the ureters

Recall that -rrhaphy means suturing. Ureter/o/rrhaphy means
*_____.

6-43

plastic surgery of the
  ureter and renal pelvis

ureter/o/pyel/itis
yōō rē′ ter ō pī ə **lī′** tis

Ureter/o/pyel/o/plasty means *_____
_____.
Form a word meaning inflammation of the ureter and renal pelvis.
_____

ANSWER COLUMN

ureter/o/cyst/o/stomy
yōō rē′ ter **ō** sis **tos′** tə mē

ureter/o/py/osis
yōō rē′ ter ō pī **ō′** sis

6-44

Form a word meaning:
making a new opening between the ureter and bladder
_____ ;

a condition of the ureter involving pus
_____ py   osis .

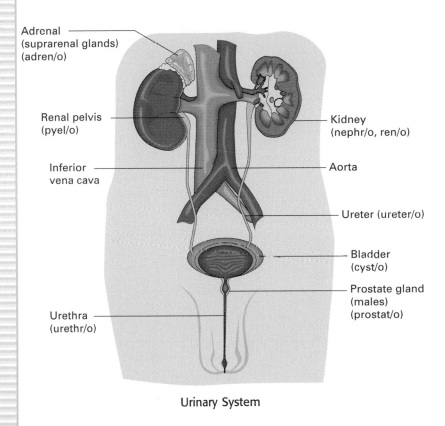

Adrenal
(suprarenal glands)
(adren/o)

Renal pelvis
(pyel/o)

Kidney
(nephr/o, ren/o)

Inferior
vena cava

Aorta

Ureter (ureter/o)

Bladder
(cyst/o)

Prostate gland
(males)
(prostat/o)

Urethra
(urethr/o)

Urinary System

6-45

Form the word that means suturing of the ureter:

ureter/o/rrhaphy
yōō rē tə **rôr′** ə fē

_____ .

ANSWER COLUMN

6-46

Form a word meaning:
suturing of a kidney

nephr/o/rrhaphy
nef **rôr′** ə fē

_____;

suturing of the bladder

cyst/o/rrhaphy
sis **tôr′** ə fē

_____.

Form a word meaning:
suture of a nerve

neur/o/rrhaphy
nŏŏ **rôr′** ə fē

_____.

6-47

The combining form for urethra is **urethr/o**.
Urethr/o/rrhaphy means

suturing of the
   urethra

*_____.

Form a word meaning:
incision into the urethra

urethr/o/tomy
yŏŏr′ ə **throt′** ə mē

_____;

spasm of the urethra

urethr/o/spasm
yŏŏ **rē′** thrō spazm

_____.

6-48

Urethr/o/rect/al means pertaining to the urethra and rectum.
Urethr/o/vagin/al means pertaining to the

urethra
yŏŏ **rē′** thrə
urethr/o/cyst/itis
yŏŏ **rē′** thrō sis tī′ tis

_____ and vagina. Form a word
that means inflammation of urethra and bladder.

_____

ANSWER COLUMN

6-49

Recall the suffix -rrhagia. Gastr/o/rrhagia means stomach hemorrhage. Encephal/o/rrhagia means brain

hem/o/rrhage
hem' o rəj
urethr/o/rrhagia
yōō rē' thrō **rā'** jē' ə

_____.

A word that means hemorrhage of the urethra is

_____.

6-50

Build a word meaning:
hemorrhage of the bladder

cyst/o/rrhagia
sis' tō **rā'** jē ə

_____;

hemorrhage of the ureter

ureter/o/rrhagia
yōō rē' ter ō **rā'** jē ə

_____.

6-51

ren/o is also used as a combining form for kidney.
Build a word meaning:
pertaining to the kidney

ren/al
rē' nəl

_____;

any kidney disease

ren/o/pathy
rē **nop'** ə thē

_____;

record from x-ray of the kidney

ren/o/gram
rē' nō gram

_____.

6-52

cyst/o is used to form words that refer to the urinary

bladder

_____.

ANSWER COLUMN

---

cyst/o

6-53

To refer to the urinary bladder, or **any sac containing fluid**, use some form of _____.

---

cyst/o/plasty
sis' tō plas' tē

6-54

A word for surgical repair of the bladder is

_____.

---

water or fluid
or
watery fluid

6-55

A hydr/o/cyst is a sac (or bladder) filled with watery fluid. **Hydr/o** is used in words to mean
* _____.

---

cyst/o/tomy
sis **tot'** ə mē

6-56

The word for incision into the bladder is

_____.

---

cyst/ectomy
sis **tek'** tə mē

6-57

The word for excision of the bladder is

_____.

6-58

Recall that -scopy is a suffix for the procedure used to look into an organ or body cavity. The process of examining by looking with an instrument into the urinary bladder is _____.

cyst/o/scopy
sis **tos'** kō pē

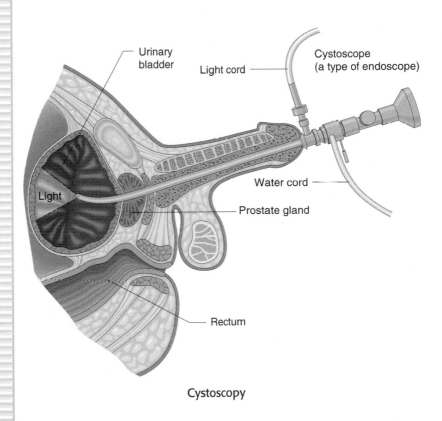

Cystoscopy

6-59

Build a word that means:
surgical repair of the bladder

_____;

cyst/o/plasty
sis' tō plas' tē

prolapse of the bladder

_____.

cyst/o/ptosis
sis top **tō'** sis

ANSWER COLUMN

6-60

When the bladder herniates into the vagina, a

cyst/o/cele
sis' tō sēl

_____ is formed.

6-61

Build a word meaning:
hemorrhage from the bladder

cyst/o/rrhagia
sis tō **rā'** jē ə

_____;

flowing from the bladder

cyst/o/rrhea
sis tō **rē'** ə

_____;

suturing of the bladder

cyst/o/rrhaphy
sis **tôr'** ə fē

_____.

Information Frame ??

6-62

Urinary dysfunction and other systemic diseases are often seen as changes in frequency of urination, character, chemistry, and inclusions in urine. Urinary tract infection (UTI), diabetes, and prostate disease are often first detected by urinary symptoms reported by a patient and signs observed by the lab technician or physician.

ANSWER COLUMN

6-63

The following table lists several common urinary symptoms and signs:

poly/uria	abnormally frequent urination
noct/uria	waking often at night to urinate
an/uria	lack of (suppression of) urine
olig/uria	abnormally low (scant) amount of urine output
hemat/uria	blood in the urine
albumin/uria	protein (albumin) in the urine
glycos/uria, glucos/uria	sugar (glucose) in the urine
keton/uria	ketones in the urine
nocturnal enuresis	bed-wetting

6-64

Using the suffix -uria (condition in the urine) build a word that means:
sugar in the urine

glycos/uria
glĭ kō **syoor'** ē ə
or glucos/uria
glōō kō **syoor'** ē ə

_____ ;

frequent urination

poly/uria
pol ē **yoor'** ē ə

_____ ;

blood in the urine

hemat/uria
hē mat **yoor'** ē ə

_____ .

6-65

Information Frame

-philia is the opposite of phobia. -phobia is abnormal fear of; -philia is abnormal or unusual attraction to.

ANSWER COLUMN

6-66

abnormal attraction
  to dead bodies

Necr/o/phobia is an abnormal fear of dead bodies.
Necr/o/philia is *_____

_____.

6-67

-phobia/-philia
hydr/o/phobia
hī drō **fō'** bē ə
hydr/o/philia
hī' drō **fil'** ē ə

hydr/o is the combining form for water. Words that can end in
-phobia can end in -philia. Morbid fear of water is

_____.

Strong attraction to water is

_____.

6-68

from

Recall that de- is a prefix. When water is taken from a substance, the
substance is less than it was.
De/hydr/ation takes water _____ something.

6-69

de/hydr/ation
dē hī **drā'** shən

When water is taken from plums, de/hydr/ation occurs, forming
prunes. When water is taken from a cell,
_____ also occurs.

6-70

de/hydr/ated
dē **hī'** drā tid

When something is dehydrated, it has less water than it did before.
When water is lost from the body because of excessive vomiting or
diarrhea, the patient is

_____.

ANSWER COLUMN

6-71

Vomiting can cause dehydration. A high fever can also

dehydration

cause _____.

6-72

Ex/cretion is the process of **ex/**pelling (or getting out from the body) a substance. Expelling urine is urinary

ex/cretion
eks **krē′** shən

_____.

6-73

Expelling carbon dioxide is respiratory

excretion

_____. Expelling sweat

excretion

is dermal _____.

6-74

excretion

Expelling menses is menstrual _____.
Expelling fecal matter is gastrointestinal

excretion

_____.

6-75

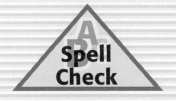

Spell Check

Excretions are usually waste substances; i.e., feces, urine. Secretions, such as hormones, are useful substances. There is a difference between excretions and secretions.

6-76

Information Frame

trans- is a prefix meaning across, as in the word transportation. Transpiration is the act of carrying water vapors across lung or skin tissue to eliminate them from the body. Breathing is respiration.

ANSWER COLUMN

6-77

Breath/ing consists of the following two processes: ex/piration and in/spiration. Think of the meaning as you analyze:

ex/pir/a/tion
eks per **ā'** shən   expiration _____;
in/spir/a/tion
in sper **ā'** shən   inspiration _____;

6-78

Build a word meaning:

ex/cise
ek **sīz'**   to cut out _____;
in/cise
in **sīz'**   to cut into _____.

6-79

Look at the words in the previous frame. The word that

inspiration   means breathing in is _____.

6-80

in- is a prefix that means in or not. In/compatible drugs

not   are drugs that do _____ mix with each other.

6-81

In/compet/ency occurs in an organ when it is

not   _____ able to perform its function.

6-82

Incompetence is a noun. Incompetent is an adjective. When the ile/o/cec/al valve cannot perform its function,

in/compet/ence   the result is ileocecal _____
in **kom'** pə təns
in/compet/ent
in **kom'** pə tənt   or an _____ ileocecal valve.

ANSWER COLUMN

	6-83
incompetence	When blood seeps back through the aortic valves, aortic _____ or insufficiency occurs.
	6-84
incompetence incompetent	When a person is not able to think rationally enough to care for himself or herself, you may call it ment/al _____ (noun). You may even say the person is mentally _____ (adjective).
	6-85
in/continence in **kon'** ti nəns	Continence is the ability to control defecation and urination. Lack of control of waste removal is called _____.
	6-86
incontinence

incontinent | "Incontinence" is a noun. "Incontinent" is an adjective. Patients with urinary _____ (noun) may wear a protective pad for clothes or bedding. The _____ (adjective) patient had a weakened urinary bladder and lost control. |
| in not

not able to be cured condition of being enclosed | **6-87** |
| | in- is a prefix that means _____ or _____.

Deduce the meaning of: incurable *_____; inclusion *_____.

Great! |

ANSWER COLUMN

The following medical abbreviations correspond to the terms in Unit 6.

Abbreviation	Meaning
ARF	acute renal failure
BPH	benign prostatic hypertrophy (hyperplasia)
BUN	blood urea nitrogen
Cysto	cystoscopy
ESRD	end-stage renal disease
GU	genitourinary
IVP	intravenous pyelogram
KUB	kidney-ureter-bladder (x-ray)
M, ♂	male
PKU	phenylketonuria
PSA	prostate specific antigen
TUR or TURP	transurethral resection of the prostate
UTI	urinary tract infection
Ua	urinalysis

You have been introduced to many new terms in this unit. To make sure you know them well, work the review exercises on the following pages. Also, listen to the CD-ROM accompanying the third edition of *Medical Terminology Made Easy* and practice pronunciation.

UNIT 6
REVIEW EXERCISE

Part 1: Review the terms you have learned in this unit by drawing the diagonal lines between the word parts and writing the meaning of each term. Use your medical dictionary or the frames if you need help. After you have completed these tasks, say each term aloud to practice pronunciation.

1. balanoplasty

2. cryptorchidism

3. cystoscopy

4. dehydration

5. excise

6. excretion

7. expiration

8. glycosuria

9. hematuria

10. hydrophilia

11. incise

12. incompetence

13. incontinence

14. inspiration

15. nephropexy

16. nephroptosis

17. nocturia

18. oliguria

19. orchidocele

20. orchidectomy

21. polyuria

22. prostatorrhea

23. pyelonephritis

24. renogram

25. spermatolysis

26. spermicide

27. ureterocystostomy

**UNIT 6
REVIEW EXERCISE**

28. ureterorrhaphy _____

29. urethrocystitis _____

30. urethrorrhagia _____

31. urology _____

32. vasectomy _____

33. vasodilatation _____

34. vasotripsy _____

Part 2: Match each term with its correct meaning.

_____ 1. spermolysis

_____ 2. balanitis

_____ 3. vasorrhaphy

_____ 4. prostatalgia

_____ 5. nephropexy

_____ 6. renal

_____ 7. cryptorchidism

_____ 8. renogram

_____ 9. urology

_____10. cystoscope

a. study of diseases of the male reproductive system and urinary system

b. inflammation of the kidney

c. x-ray of the kidney

d. discharge from the penis

e. prolapse of the urethra

f. inflammation of the penis

g. suturing of the vas deferens

h. tumor of the prostate gland

i. instrument used to look into the kidney

j. hidden testicle

k. adjective for kidney

l. prostatic pain

m. fixation of prolapsed kidney

n. instrument used to look into the bladder

o. destruction of sperm

Part 3: Write the medical term that means:

1. inflammation of the tube that leads from the bladder to the outside of the body_____

2. hemorrhage of the urinary bladder _____

3. waking to urinate at night_____

4. inflammation of the kidney tissue and renal pelvis_____

UNIT 6
REVIEW EXERCISE

5. dilation of a vessel _____

6. suturing of the tube that leads from the kidney to the bladder _____

7. herniation of the testicle_____

8. prolapse of a kidney_____

9. inability to control urination _____

10. loss of fluid from the body _____

Part 4: Use the medical terms listed below to complete these sentences:

vasectomy	testicular	hydrophobia	dehydrated	prostatic
excise	incision	ureterolith	BPH	urologist
incompetent	cystorrhagia	pyelogram	orchidoplasty	

1. The _____ instructed the male patient about performing _____ self-exam for early detection of cancer.

2. A slow urine stream and difficulty in urinating prompted the doctor to examine Mr. Elder for prostate disease. The prostate was enlarged but not cancerous, indicating a diagnosis of benign _____ hypertrophy (Abbrev. _____).

3. Mr. S. I. Hurtz complained of extreme left quadrant and lumbar pain. An intravenous _____ was performed, showing a stone in the ureter called a _____.

4. Sheila Thurston had the flu. For three days she vomited and had diarrhea. Her skin was dry and it was necessary to put her on IV therapy because she was _____.

5. A three centimeter _____ was made in order to _____ the lesion.

6. Blood in the urine and cystoscopic exam revealed an injury to the bladder, causing _____.

7. Rabies causes end-stage symptoms of madness characterized by fear of water. That is why rabies is also called _____.

8. Dr. B. Steral ordered a sperm count after surgery to determine the success of the _____ procedure.

UNIT 6
REVIEW EXERCISE

Part 5: Draw a line to match the abbreviation with its meaning.

1. ESRD   blood urea nitrogen

2. KUB   cystoscopy

3. PKU   end stage renal disease

4. UTI   urinary tract infection

5. M, ♂   phenylketonuria

6. Cysto   male

7. IVP   kidney, ureter, bladder x-ray

8. BUN   intravenous pyelogram

**UNIT 6
REVIEW EXERCISE**

Part 6: Label the structures of the urinary and male reproductive systems. Then draw a line to the combining form matching the structure.

1. rect/o   _____

2. cyst/o   _____

3. urethr/o   _____

4. balan/o   _____

5. prostat/o   _____

6. vas/o   _____

7. orchid/o   _____

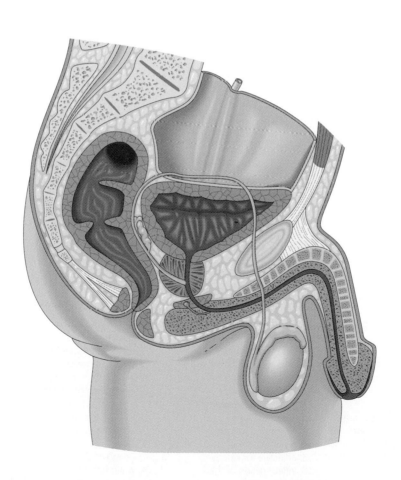

Unit 6 Puzzle

As a self-test work the crossword puzzle and then check your answers in Appendix F.

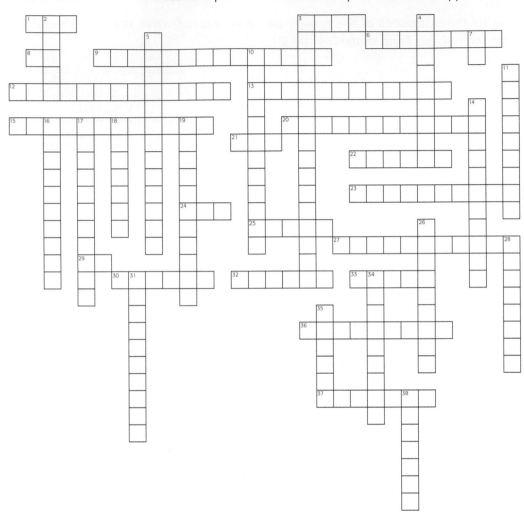

ACROSS

1. benign prostatic hyperplasia (abbrev.)
3. combining form for vessel
6. abnormally frequent urination
8. prefix for down from or less than normal
9. hidden testicle
12. discharge from the prostate
13. surgery to remove the foreskin around the penis
15. suture of the bladder
20. not competent
21. urinary tract infection (abbrev.)
22. tube from the kidney to the bladder
23. sugar in the urine
24. prostate specific antigen
25. cystoscopy (abbrev.)
27. breath in
29. genitourinary (abbrev.)
30. suffix for fear
32. combining form for glans penis
33. adjective for kidney
36. inflammation of the kidney tissue
37. sack containing the testes

DOWN

2. combining form for renal pelvis
3. condition of making the vessel diameter smaller
4. hernation of the bladder
5. destruction of sperm
7. prefix for not or in
10. inability to control urination or defecation
11. I.V. _____ (x-ray)
14. water has been taken away from the body
16. agent that destroys sperm
17. testicular pain
18. suffix for suturing
19. attraction to water
26. specialist in urinary system disorders
28. waking to urinate at night
31. bleed
34. process of expelling waste
35. plural for more than one testis
38. tube from the bladder to the outside

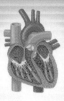

UNIT 7
Female Reproductive System, Obstetrics, and Neonatology

Study these word parts, meanings, and examples. Then proceed to the first frame.

COMBINING FORMS

amni/o (amnion)
cervic/o (cervix, neck)
colp/o (vagina)
gravid/o (pregnant woman)
gynec/o (woman)
hyster/o (uterus)
lapar/o (abdomen)
mamm/o (mammary glands)
mast/o (breast)
men/o (menstruation)
metr/o (uterine tissues)
nat/o (birth)
o/o (egg, ovum)
oophor/o (ovary)
salping/o (uterine tube)
syphil/o (syphilis)
top/o (place)
vagin/o (vagina)

PREFIXES

a– (without, lack of)
aniso– (unequal)
ante– (before)
bi– (two, both)
dys– (difficult, painful)
ecto– (outside of)

endo– (inner)
infra– (below, under)
iso– (same, equal)
multi– (many)
neo– (new)
nulli– (none)
post– (after)
pre– (before, in front of)
primi– (first)

SUFFIXES

–blast (immature or embryonic cell)
–centesis (surgical puncture for fluid removal)
–ectopic (out of place)
–graphy (process of making a picture or record)
–gravida (pregnancy)
–para (woman who carries pregnancy to viability)
–partum (delivery, childbirth)
–pexy (fixation of a prolapse)
–phobia (fear)
–ptosis (prolapse)
–scope (instrument used to look)
–scopy (process of using a scope)
–stasis (control or stopping)

Word Examples

COMBINING FORMS
amniocentesis
cervical
colpodynia
primigravida
gynecology
hysteroscope
laparotomy
mammogram
mastectomy
menorrhea
metrorrhagia
natal
oogenesis
oophoritis
salpingocele
syphilis
ectopic
vaginal

PREFIXES
amenorrhea
anisomastia
antepartum
bilateral

dystocia
ectopic
endometrium
inframammary
isotonic
multiparous
neonatal
nullipara
postpartum
prenatal
primiparous

SUFFIXES
ooblast
amniocentesis
mammography
nulligravida
multipara
prepartum
oophoropexy
syphilophobia
hysteroptosis
hysteroscope
laparoscopy
menostasis

ANSWER COLUMN

7-1

The Greek word for egg is "oon." In scientific words, **o/o** (pronounced ō/ə, or ōō, or ō/o) means egg or ovum. An o/o/blast is * _____ .

an embryonic egg cell
(a cell that will
become an ovum)

7-2

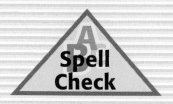

Spell
Check

"Ova" is plural and "ovum" is singular for eggs and egg. Ovular is the adjectival form.

7-3

o/o/genesis
ō′ ə **jen′** ə sis

Oogenesis is the formation and development of an ovum. The changes that occur in the cell from ooblast to mature ovum are _____ .

7-4

ov/ulation
ov yōō **lā′** shən

Oogenesis must be complete for the ovum to be mature. Then ovulation (the release of the mature egg) can occur. The release of an ovum from the ovary is _____ .

7-5

ovary

The combining form used in words that refer to the ovary is **oophor/o**. This literally means "egg **(o/o)** bearing **(phor/o)**." When you see **oophor** in a word, you think of the _____ .

ANSWER COLUMN

7-6

The ovary is the organ responsible for maturing and discharging the ovum. About every 28 days ovulation occurs. An ovum is discharged from the _____.

ovary

7-7

This frame shows the development of oophorectomy:

o/o		egg	from Greek, oon
	phor/o	bear	from Greek, phoros
	ect/o	out	from Greek, ektos
	tomy	cut	from Greek, tomos

This is included for those who are interested.

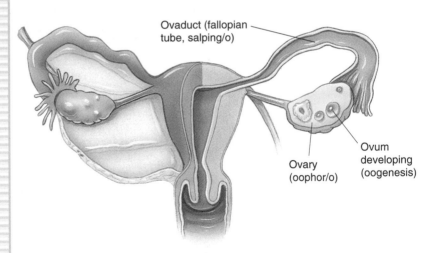

Ovaduct (fallopian tube, salping/o)

Ovum developing (oogenesis)

Ovary (oophor/o)

Ovulation

ANSWER COLUMN

oophor/itis or
ō of′ ō **ri′** tis
ōō fō **ri′** tis

oophor/ectomy or
ō of′ ō **rek′** tə me
ōō fō **rek′** tə me

oophor/oma or
ō of′ ō **rō** mə
ōō fō **rō** mə

7-8

Using what you need from **oophor/o**, build a word that means:
inflammation of an ovary

_____;

excision of an ovary

_____;

tumor of an ovary
(ovarian tumor)

_____.

7-9

Sometimes an organ becomes prolapsed because the support
tissues get stretched. Oophor/o/ptosis is a prolapsed (dropped
or sagged) ovary. The suffix for prolapsed is

–ptosis

_____. (More on this later.)

7-10

fixation

orchi/o/pexy
ôr′ kē ō pek′ sē or
orchid/o/pexy
ôr′ kid ō pek sē
nephr/o/pexy
nef′ rō pek sē

Oophor/o/pexy means fixation of a displaced or prolapsed ovary.
-pexy is a suffix that means

_____.

Fixation of a displaced testicle is

_____;

Fixation of a displaced kidney is

_____.

ANSWER COLUMN

7-11

salping/o is used to build words that refer to the uterine tubes. A salping/o/scope is an instrument used to examine the

uterine tube(s)

*_____.

7-12

A salping/o/stomy is a surgical opening into a

uterine tube

*_____.

7-13

Using what you need of **salping/o**, build a word meaning: inflammation of a uterine tube

salping/itis
sal′ pin **jī′** tis

_____;

excision of a uterine tube

salping/ectomy
sal′ pin **jek′** tə mē

_____.

7-14

When you are building compound medical words and use two like vowels between word roots or combining forms, separate them with a hyphen. For a model use **salping/o-oophor/ectomy** and build a word that means inflammation of the fallopian tube and ovary.

salping/o-/oophor/itis
sal pin′ gō ō of′ ō **rī′** tis

_____-_____

7-15

A hernia that encloses the uterine (fallopian) tube and ovary is a

salping/o-/oophor/o/cele
sal ping′ gō ō **of′** or ō sēl

_____-_____.

ANSWER COLUMN

7-16

colp/o is used in words about the vagina. Colp/itis

inflammation of
the vagina

means *_____.

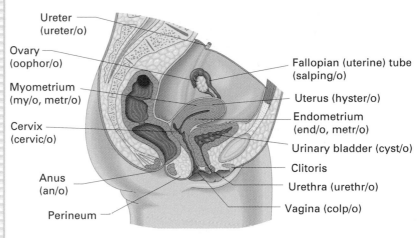

Ureter
(ureter/o)

Ovary
(oophor/o)

Myometrium
(my/o, metr/o)

Cervix
(cervic/o)

Anus
(an/o)

Perineum

Fallopian (uterine) tube
(salping/o)

Uterus (hyster/o)

Endometrium
(end/o, metr/o)

Urinary bladder (cyst/o)

Clitoris

Urethra (urethr/o)

Vagina (colp/o)

Female Reproductive System

7-17

vaginal pain

Colp/o/dynia means *_____.
Suture of the vagina is called

colp/o/rrhaphy
kol **por′** ə fē

_____.

7-18

vaginal spasm

Colp/o/spasm is a *_____.
Excision of a part of the vagina is a

colp/ectomy
kol **pek′** tə mē

_____.

7-19

Build a word meaning:
fixation of a prolapsed vagina

colp/o/pexy
kol' pō pek sē

_____ ;

surgical repair of the vagina

colp/o/plasty
kol' pō plas' tē

_____ .

7-20

Build a word meaning:
instrument for examining the vagina

colp/o/scope
kol' pō skōp

_____ ;

process of examining the vagina with a scope

colp/o/scopy
kol **pos'** ko pē

_____ .

7-21

hyster/o is used to build words about the uterus as an organ.
A hyster/ectomy is an excision of the

uterus
yōō' ter əs

_____ .

7-22

A hyster/o/tomy is an incision into the

uterus
uterus

_____ , and a hyster/o/spasm
is a spasm of the _____ .

ANSWER COLUMN

7-23

A hyster/o/gram is an x-ray (picture) of the uterus.
A general term for any disease of the uterus is:

hyster/o/pathy
his′ ter **op′** ə thē

_____.

A hyster/o/scope is used to look inside the

uterus

_____.

NOTE: See illustration on pg 255.

7-24

There is a special x-ray procedure performed to determine patency
(openness) of the fallopian tubes by injecting a contrast medium.
This "picture" of the uterus and uterine tubes is called a:

hyster/o/salping/o/gram
his′ ter ō sal
        pin′ gō gram

_____ (HSG).

7-25

A hyster/o/salping/o-/oophor/ectomy is the excision of the uterus,
fallopian tubes, and ovaries. Analyze this word:

hyster/o
salping/o
oophor
ectomy

_____	combining form for uterus
_____	combining form for fallopian tubes
_____	word root for ovary
_____	suffix—excision

7-26

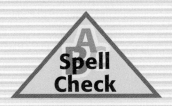

Watch for the hyphen when three "o's" are together, as in salpingo-
oophorectomy or salpingo-oophoritis.

7-27

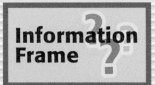

hyster/o is used in words pertaining to the uterus as an organ.
metr/o refers to the tissue layers of the uterus.

ANSWER COLUMN

7-28

hyster/o usually refers to the uterus as a whole organ.
metr/o usually refers to the tissues or layers of the

uterus

_____.

7-29

organ

There are exceptions to the rule, but generally **hyster/o**
means the uterus as an _____.
Metr/o refers to the uterus in the sense of its

tissues

_____.

7-30

Metr/itis means an inflammation of the uterine musculature or
my/o/met/rium. Metr/o/paralysis means paralysis of the

uterus or
uterine musculature

* _____.

7-31

Using **metr/o** and rrhea, build a word meaning flow or discharge
from the uterine tissues _____.

metr/o/rrhea
mē trō **rē′** ə

7-32

Build a word meaning:
any uterine disease

metr/o/pathy
mē **trop′** ə thē or
hyster/o/pathy
his ter **op′** ə thē
metr/o/cele
mē′ trō sēl or
hyster/o/cele
his′ ter ō sēl

_____;

herniation of the uterus

_____.

ANSWER COLUMN

7-33

The end/o/metr/ium is the inner lining of the uterus. Build a word meaning:

inflammation of the inner uterine lining

_____;

endo/metr/itis
en' dō mə **trī'** tis

condition of the uterine tissue

_____.

endo/metri/osis
en' dō mē trē **ō'** sis

7-34

Build the word that means excision of the uterus, fallopian tubes, and ovaries.

_____ - _____

hyster/o/salping/o-/
  oophor/ectomy
his' ter ō sal pin' gō ō' of
  or **ek'** tə mē

_____.

7-35

Recall that -ptosis is a suffix. Hyster/o/ptosis means prolapse of the uterus. -Ptosis is a word and suffix that means

prolapse, or downward
  displacement

*_____.

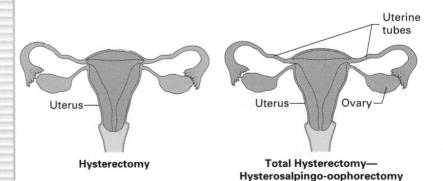

Uterine
tubes

Uterus

Hysterectomy

Uterus   Ovary

**Total Hysterectomy—
Hysterosalpingo-oophorectomy**

ANSWER COLUMN

7-36

Hyster/o/ptosis is a compound word constructed from:

hyster/o

ptosis

_____ the combining form for uterus;

_____ a suffix meaning prolapse.

7-37

When prolapse occurs, a fixation is usually done. A hysteropexy would be done to correct or fixate

hyster/o/ptosis
his′ ter op **tō′** sis

_____.

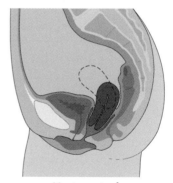

Hysteroptosis

7-38

Build a word meaning prolapse of the vagina:

colp/o/ptosis
kol′ pop **tō′** sis

_____.

7-39

A word meaning surgical fixation of the uterus is

hyster/o/pex/y
his′ ter ō pek sē

_____.

A word meaning uterine hernia is

hyster/o/cele
his′ ter ō sēl

_____.

ANSWER COLUMN

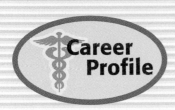

obstetr/ician
ob ste **tri'** shən

7-40

The physician specialist who gives prenatal care and facilitates the delivery of babies is called an **obstetrician** (OB). An

_____ specializes in delivery of babies and care of the mother during the birth process.

---

obstetrics
ob **ste'** trikz

7-41

Obstetrics is the specialty that studies and works with women who are pregnant or giving birth.
The obstetrician practices

_____.

---

women

7-42

gynec/o comes from the Greek word "gyne," which means woman. The field of medicine called gynecology
deals with diseases of _____.

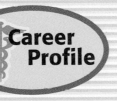

gynec/o/log/ist
gī nə **kol'** ə jist,
jin ə **kol'** ə jist

7-43

Gynec/o/log/ic or gynec/o/log/ical are adjectival forms of gynec/o/logy. The physician who specializes in female disorders is called a _____ (GYN).

7-44

Build a word meaning:
resembling woman

_____;

gynec/oid
gī′ nə koid

any disease peculiar to women

_____;

gynec/o/pathy
gī′ nə **kop′** ə thē

abnormal fear of women

_____.

gynec/o/phobia
gī′ ne kō **fō′** bē ə

Information Frame

7-45

cervic/o can mean the neck as well as the neck of the uterus. In usage you are not likely to confuse them. A person injured in an auto accident might be required to wear a cervical collar. Cervical dilation occurs during labor.

7-46

Cervic/o is the combining form for cervix. **Cervic** is the word root. Build a word meaning:
excision of the cervix

_____;

cervic/ectomy
ser vi **sek′** tə mē

inflammation of the cervix

_____;

cervic/itis
ser vi **sī′** tis

pertaining to the cervix

_____.

cervic/al
ser′ vi kəl

ANSWER COLUMN

abdominal wall

7-47

lapar/o means abdominal wall. A laparocele is a herniation of the *_____.

lapar/o/scopy
lap ə **ros'** kō pē

7-48

Process of examining the abdominal cavity with a laparoscope is called _____.

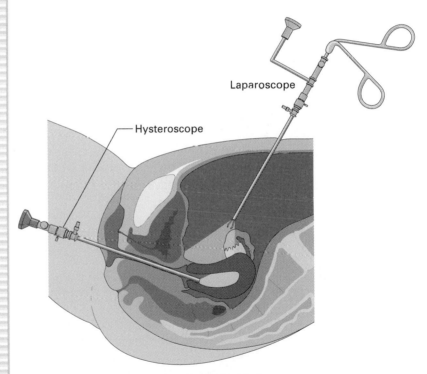

Laparoscope

Hysteroscope

Laparoscopy performed with hysteroscopy

lapar/o/tomy
lap ə **rot'** ə mē
lapar/o/rrhaphy
lap ə **rôr'** ə fē

7-49

An incision into the abdominal wall is a
_____.

A suturing of the abdominal wall is
_____.

ANSWER COLUMN

7-50

Laparoscopically assisted vaginal hysterectomy (LAVH)
makes use of a _____.

laparoscope
lap' ər ō skōp

7-51

There may be longer words than this. If there are, there are not
many. Analyze it for fun. Think of the word parts.
Laparohysterosalpingo-oophorectomy *_____

abdomen,
uterus, uterine tubes,
    ovaries, excision

_____.

7-52

Centesis is a surgical puncture usually done with a needle and
tubing to remove fluid from a body cavity. Thorac/o/centesis is the
surgical puncture or tapping of the chest. Build a word that would
mean a surgical puncture of the following cavities:
abdominal

abdomin/o/centesis   abdomin   o _____ ;
ab dom' i nō sen **tē'** sis

pleura
pleur/o/centesis   pleur   o _____ .
ploor' ō sen **tē** sis

7-53

If bleeding in the chest cavity is suspected, a surgical tap
of the chest, or _____, may be done.

thorac/o/centesis
thor' a kō sen **tē'** sis

7-54

If fluid from cancer cells is building up in the abdomen,
an _____ may be
abdomin/o/centesis   done to remove the fluid.
NOTE: This is also called paracentesis.

ANSWER COLUMN

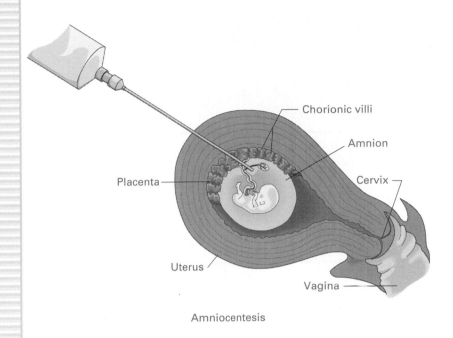

Chorionic villi

Amnion

Cervix

Placenta

Uterus

Vagina

Amniocentesis

7-55

iso- is used as a prefix to mean equal or the same. Something that is ɪso/metɪ/ic is of _____ _____ dimensions.

equal

7-56

Iso/cyt/o/sis is a condition in which cells are of _____ size.

equal

7-57

An isotonic solution has the same osmotic pressure as red blood cells. Normal saline is an _____ solution.

iso/ton/ic
ī sō **ton'** ik

7-58

Intra/ven/ous ringers lactate is another _____ solution.

isotonic

ANSWER COLUMN

7-59

iso- is a prefix for equal. an- is a prefix meaning without.
Something that is without equality is unequal.

aniso- or aniso

The prefix for unequal is _____.

7-60

Mastos is the Greek word for breast. Mastia is a condition

breast

of the _____.
Aniso/mastia means that a woman's breasts are of

unequal

_____ size.

7-61

Inflammation of the breast is mast/itis. Surgical excision of part or all

mast/ectomy
mas **tek'** tə mē

of the breast is a _____.

7-62

Build a term that means a cancerous tumor of the breast:

mast/o/carcin/oma
mas' tō kar sin **ō'** mə

_____.

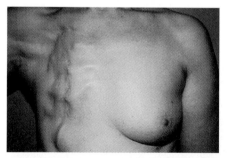

Radical mastectomy patient
(*Photo courtesy of Steven M. Lynh, M.D.*)

ANSWER COLUMN

aniso/cyt/osis
an ī′ sō sī **tō′** sis

anisocytosis

anisocytosis

mamm/o/graphy
mam **og′** ra fē

7-63

Anis/o/cyt/osis means that cells are of unequal sizes. This word is commonly limited to a condition of red blood cells in medical diagnosis. A word indicating a condition of inequality in cell size is

_____.

7-64

Normal red blood cells are the same size (7.2 microns). An anemic condition resulting in unequal size of red blood cells is _____.

7-65

Red blood cells are formed in the bone marrow. An unhealthy bone marrow can result in unequal red blood cells, or

_____.

7-66

mamm/o is another combining form for breast. An x-ray picture of the breast is a mammogram or mammograph. The process of taking this x-ray is called

_____.

NOTE: Mammography is an important procedure for early detection of breast cancer.

ANSWER COLUMN

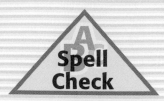

7-67

Notice the correct spelling and pronunciation of the word mammogram. It is pronounced **mam'** ō gram, **not** mammiogram, (**mam'** ē ō gram), as many people do.

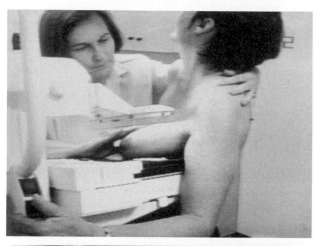

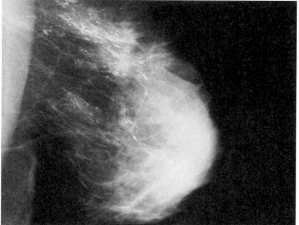

Mammography (*top*) Positioning for Cleopatra view;
(*bottom*) Cleopatra view radiograph

7-68

Augmentation of the breast to increase the volume may be done following a mastectomy for treatment of breast cancer. This surgical repair of the breast is

_____.

mamm/o/plasty
mam' ō plas tē

ANSWER COLUMN

7-69

If the breast is too large, then a reduction

mammoplasty

_____ may be performed.

7-70

Whenever a procedure is performed on both sides, it is said to be "bilateral." A bilateral hernia repair is on

both sides   *_____. A bilateral mammogram is
both breasts   a radiograph of *_____.

7-71

Infra- means below or under. Infra/mammary means

below or under   *_____ the mammary gland.

7-72

men/o is used in words referring to the menses. Men/ses is another way of saying men/struation. **men/o** in any word should make you

men/ses   think of _____.
men′ sĕz or
men/struation
men strōō **ā′** shən

7-73

Men/o/pause means permanent cessation of

menstruation or menses   *_____.
excessive menstruation   Men/o/rrhagia means *_____.
  occuring at irregular   (Pronounced: **men′** ō paws, men ō **rā′** jē ə)
  intervals or menstrual
  hemorrhage

ANSWER COLUMN

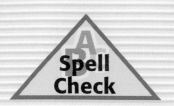

Spell Check

7-74

"Menstruation" and "menstrual" are often misspelled by leaving out the "u." You should also remember to pronounce the "u" as men strōō **ā'** shən and **men'** strōō əl.

7-75

Men/arche refers to a female's first menstrual period. Menarche (**men'** ar kē) comes from the Greek words **"men"** for month and **"arche"** for beginning. Build a word meaning:
flow of menses

menstruation or
men/o/rrhea
men ō **rē'** ə

_____ ;

painful (bad or difficult) menstrual flow

dys/men/o/rrhea
dis men ō **rē'** ə

_____ .

7-76

Build a word meaning:
absence (without) of menstrual flow

a/men/o/rrhea
ā men ō **rē'** ə

_____ ;

stopping menstrual flow (by medication or surgery)

men/o/stasis
ā men ō **rē'** ə
mə **nos'** te sis or
    men ō **stā** sis

_____ .

Information Frame

7-77

dys- is the prefix for painful, faulty, diseased, bad, or difficult. **men** is the word root for menstruation.

ANSWER COLUMN

dys/men/o/rrhea
dis men ō **rē′** ə

7-78

Painful or difficult menstruation is

_____.

7-79

Information Frame ??

Many women experience a series of symptoms prior to the onset of menstruation. This premenstrual syndrome (PMS) may include headaches, water retention, breast soreness, anxiety and tension increase, appetite increase, and fatigue. It may have a duration of several days to two weeks and is relieved by the onset of menstruation.

7-80

multi
many or
   more than one

multi- is a prefix for many or more than one. You are acquainted with multi- in the words multiply and multitude. Something composed of multiple parts or numbers uses
_____ as a prefix. Multi/gravida refers to a woman having _____ pregnancies.

7-81

many glands

many cells

many nuclei

Multi/glandular is an adjective meaning
*_____.
Multi/cellular is an adjective meaning
*_____.
Multi/nuclear is an adjective meaning
*_____.

ANSWER COLUMN

multi/para
mul **tip'** ə rə

7-82

A multi/para is a woman who has brought forth (borne) more than one child. para- is a Latin suffix meaning to bear a viable fetus. Multi/par/ous is the adjectival form of

_____.

Pronunciation note: Notice multipara has the primary accent on **tip'**. It is pronounced mul **tip'** ərə, not mul tē **par'a**.

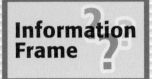

7-83

The suffix -para is used when referring to viable births or potentially viable births weighing 500 grams or more or occurring after the 20th week of pregnancy. Termination of pregnancies of less than 500 grams or 20 weeks by either accidental, tubal, induced, or spontaneous abortion (miscarriage) are listed as abortions (Ab), i.e., Para II , Ab I, Grav III.

---

multipara

7-84

Multi/para **always** refers to the mother. Multi/par/ous may refer to the mother or may mean multiple birth (twins or triplets). When desiring to indicate that a woman has borne more than one child, use the noun _____.

---

multipara
multi/parous
mul **tip'** ar əs

7-85

"Multiparous" is the adjectival form of

_____. To indicate that twins are born, say a _____ birth.

NOTE: If these are the only two viable births for this mother, the chart will say Para II.

ANSWER COLUMN

7-86

To indicate that triplets are born, say _____

multiparous

multiparous

birth. If ten children are born, you would still use the adjective

_____.

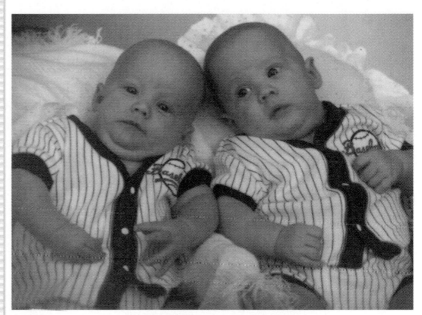

Identical twins: multiparous

(refers to a woman who has given birth to more than one child)

7-87

nulli- means none. To nullify something is to bring it to nothing.

There are not many medical words using nulli, but when

you see it, it means _____.

7-88

a woman who has
  never borne a child

primi/para

prī **mip′** a rə

A nulli/para is *_____. Primi-

means first. A woman who is having her first labor and

delivery is a _____ (noun).

ANSWER COLUMN

7-89

"Gravida" is a Latin word meaning pregnant woman. A woman experiencing her first pregnancy is called a

primi/gravida
prīm i **grav'** i da
multi-gravida
mul tē **grav'** ida

_____ (Grav I).
A woman who has experienced two or more pregnancies is called _____.

7-90

gravida refers to pregnancies. A woman who has been pregnant four times and had two spontaneous abortions (miscarriages) and two viable births would be described on the chart as Grav IV, Ab II, Para II. The word part used for pregnancy

gravida
grav' i da

is _____.

7-91

Analyze the following and define.

nulli/para
nu **lip'** a rə
no viable (live) births
nulli/par/ous
nu **lip'** a rəs
pertaining to no
viable (live) births
primi/para
prī **mip'** a rə
first (live) birth
multi/para
mul **tip'** är a
many viable (live) births

nullipara _____ (noun)
* _____

nulliparous _____ (adjective)
* _____

primipara _____ (noun)
* _____

multipara_____ (noun)
* _____

ANSWER COLUMN

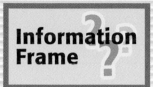

Information Frame

7-92

Note the involved development of the word "ectopic"
(out of place):
ect/o—outside
top/o—place (combining form)
   ic—adjectival suffix

7-93

ec/topic
ek **top'** ik

An ec/topic pregnancy occurs outside of the uterus (usually in a uterine [fallopian] tube). A salping/ectomy may be required after the rupture of an _____ pregnancy.

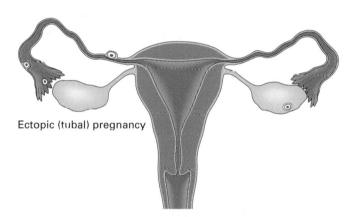

Ectopic (tubal) pregnancy

7-94

ectopic

If endometrial tissue occurs in the uterine (fallopian) tubes, a fertilized egg can lodge in it, thus causing pregnancy.
This is an _____ pregnancy.

7-95

ectopic

An embryo's development in the abdominal cavity is also an _____ pregnancy.

ANSWER COLUMN

7-96

pre- is a prefix meaning before or in front of.

before

in front of

Pre/an/esthetic means _____

anesthesia. Pre/molar means * _____

the permanent first molars.

7-97

ante- is another prefix meaning before, in front of, or forward.

before

forward

Ante/pyretic means _____ the fever.

Ante/flexion means _____ bending.

7-98

post/nat/al

pōst **nā′** təl

pre/nat/al

prē **nā′** təl

ante/nat/al

an tē **nā′** təl

Nat/al means birth. Think of the meaning while you analyze:

postnatal _____;

prenatal _____;

antenatal _____.

7-99

post- is a prefix meaning after.

Febr/ile means pertaining to fever. Build a word meaning:

pertaining to after a fever

post/febr/ile

post **fe′** brəl

_____;

pertaining to before a fever

ante/febr/ile

an′ tē **fe′** brəl

_____.

ANSWER COLUMN

7-100

Build a word meaning pertaining to:
after an operation

post/operative
pōst **op'** er ə tiv

_____ operative;

after coitus (intercourse)

post/coit/al
pōst **kō'** it əl

_____ coit _____ al;

after delivery (refers to the mother)

post/partum
pōst **par'** tum

_____ partum;

after birth (refers to the baby)

post/natal
pōst **nā** təl

_____ .

7-101

Information Frame ?

The **puerperium** is a term used to refer to the time, about three to six weeks, following birth in which the mother physically recovers from pregnancy and giving birth. The word comes from two Latin words "_puer_," meaning child, and "_parere_," to bring forth or bear. And so the **puerperium** is the time after bearing a child.

7-102

A term similar to post/partum that means after giving birth is

puer/perium
pyōōr **pair'** ē əm

_____ .

7-103

Maternal complications such as uterine infection or bleeding that develop in the puerperial period happen during the time

after giving birth

* _____ .

ANSWER COLUMN

7-104

neo- means new. From what you now know about natal, write the meaning of the term neo/nat/al:

pertaining to the
new born

*_____.

The specialty that studies treatment of newborns is

ne/o/nat/o/logy

_____.

7-105

Natal refers to birth and terms related to the newborn baby. **Partum** refers to delivery and terms related to the mother. Neonatology is the specialty that studies _____.

newborns

7-106

Use pre- to build a word (adjective) that means:
before an operation

pre/operative

_____;

before maturity (readiness)

pre/mature

_____;

in front of the frontal lobe of the brain

pre/frontal

_____;

before cancer develops

pre/cancerous
(You pronounce)

_____.

7-107

Mortem means death. What do these terms mean?

after death   postmortem *_____

before death   antemortem *_____

7-108

Syphilis is a sexually transmitted infection. Read about this in your dictionary. Note the origin of the word. Look at the words beginning with **syphil**. The combining form used in words referring to this disease is _____.

syphil/o

7-109

Using **syphil**, build terms that mean:
fear of contracting syphilis

_____;

syphil/o/phobia
sif i lō **fō′** bē ə

therapy for syphilis

_____.

syphil/o/therapy
sif i lō **ther′** ə pē

7-110

Build a word meaning:
a syphilitic tumor

_____;

syphil/oma

any syphilitic disease

_____.

syphil/o/pathy
(You pronounce)

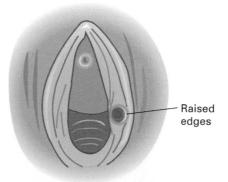

Raised edges

Syphilitic Chancre

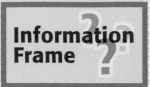

Information Frame

7-111

Other STIs (sexually transmitted infections) are more prevalent than syphilis. These include herpes simplex II, gonorrhea, HIV (human immunodeficiency virus), chlamydiae, and human papilloma virus (HPV). Some of these are presented in Unit 10.

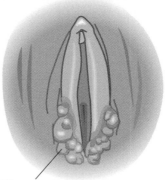

Warts caused by
human papillomavirus (HPV)

The following medical abbreviations correspond to the terms in Unit 7.

Abbreviation	Meaning
Ab I, II, III, and so on	one abortion, two, three, and so on
C-section	cesarean section delivery
D&C	dilation and curettage
F, ♀	female
FTT	failure to thrive
Grav I, II, III, and so on	one pregnancy, two, three, and so on
GYN	gynecology
HPV	human papilloma virus
HSG	hysterosalpingogram
IUD	intrauterine device
LAVH	laparoscopically assisted vaginal hysterectomy
LMP	last menstrual period
OB	obstetrics
Pap	Papanicolaou test (smear)
Para I, II, III, and so on	one live birth, two, three, and so on
PMS	premenstrual syndrome
preg	pregnant
RPR	syphilis test (also VDRL, STS, RPR)
SIDS	sudden infant death syndrome
STI or STD	sexually transmitted infection (disease)

You have been introduced to many new terms in this unit. To make sure you know them well, work the review exercises on the following pages. Also, listen to the CD-ROM accompanying the third edition of *Medical Terminology Made Easy* and practice pronunciation.

**UNIT 7
REVIEW EXERCISE**

Part 1: Review the terms you have learned in this unit by drawing the diagonal lines between the word parts and writing the meaning of each term. Use your medical dictionary or the frames if you need help. After you have completed these tasks, say each term aloud to practice pronunciation.

1. anisocytosis _____

2. anisomastia _____

3. antepartum _____

4. cervicitis _____

5. colpoplasty _____

6. colposcopy _____

7. dysmenorrhea _____

8. ectopic _____

9. endometritis _____

10. gynecologist _____

11. hysteropexy _____

12. hysteroptosis _____

13. hysterosalpingogram _____

14. hysterosalpingo-oophorectomy _____

15. inframammary _____

16. laparorrhaphy _____

17. laparoscope _____

18. mammography _____

19. mastectomy _____

20. menopause _____

21. menstruation _____

22. metrorrhea _____

23. multiparous _____

24. neonatal _____

25. nullipara _____

26. obstetrician _____

27. obstetrics _____

28. oogenesis   _____

29. oophorectomy   _____

30. oophoropexy   _____

31. postfebrile   _____

32. postmortem   _____

33. postpartum   _____

34. prenatal   _____

35. preoperative   _____

36. primigravida   _____

37. puerperium   _____

38. salpingo-oophoritis   _____

39. salpingoscope   _____

40. syphilopsychosis   _____

Part 2: Match each term with its correct meaning.

_____ 1. ooblast

_____ 2. oophoropexy

_____ 3. salpingocele

_____ 4. colporrhaphy

_____ 5. hysterosalpingogram

_____ 6. hysteroptosis

_____ 7. laparoscopy

_____ 8. mastectomy

_____ 9. metrorrhagia

_____ 10. amenorrhea

a. difficult or painful menstruation

b. excision of the breast

c. prolapse of the uterus

d. hemorrhage of the uterine tissues

e. absence of menstruation

f. embryonic egg cell

g. surgical fixation of the ovaries

h. excision of the ovaries

i. menopause

j. prolapse or sagging of the abdomen

k. process of examining the abdomen

l. herniation of the uterine tube

m. fixation of a prolapsed ovary

n. suture of the vagina

o. x-ray of the uterus and uterine tubes

UNIT 7
REVIEW EXERCISE

Part 3: Write the medical term that means:

1. cancer of the breast _____

2. x-ray picture of the breast _____

3. unequal size cells _____

4. before birth _____

5. physician specialist in womens' health _____

6. the first pregnancy _____

7. no live births _____

8. fear of syphilis _____

9. process of taking a breast x-ray _____

10. pregnancy outside of the uterus _____

Part 4: Use the medical terms listed below to complete these sentences:

multigravida	bipara	mammogram	hysteroptosis	ova
oophoroma	anisomastia	menstruation	hysteroscope	ovum
colposcopy	endometriosis	ovulation	mammoplasty	aborted
dysmenorrhea	syphilopsychosis	hysteropexy		

1. The chart notes indicated a history including: Grav V, Para II, and Ab III. This patient had many pregnancies, so she could be called a _____. However, she spontaneously _____ three times and then had two viable births, otherwise called _____.

2. One breast was much larger than the other. The condition is called _____, for which a reduction _____ was performed.

3. Upon laparoscopic examination, endometrial tissue was seen on the outside of the uterus, which confirmed the diagnosis of _____.

4. Endometrial ablation was performed while looking through a _____.

5. After many years of not being treated the syphilis spread to the brain, causing a severe mental condition called _____.

6. Once a month in the ovary the release of an _____ occurs during _____.

UNIT 7
REVIEW EXERCISE

Part 5: Draw a line to match the abbreviation with its meaning.

1. D&C   premenstrual syndrome

2. FTT   female

3. OB   one viable birth

4. HSG   dilation and curettage

5. Pap   failure to thrive

6. PMS   hysterosalpingogram

7. F ♀   obstetrics

8. Para I   Papanicolaou test

UNIT 7
REVIEW EXERCISE

Part 6: Label the structures of the female reproductive system. Then draw a line to the combining form that matches the structure.

1. colp/o   _____

2. hyster/o   _____

3. oophor/o   _____

4. metr/o   _____

5. salping/o   _____

6. cervic/o   _____

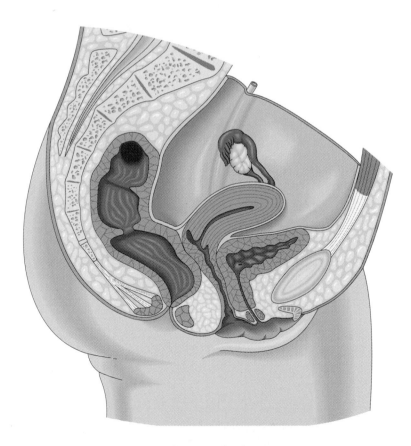

Female Reproductive System

Unit 7 Puzzle

As a self-test work the crossword puzzle and then check your answers in Appendix F.

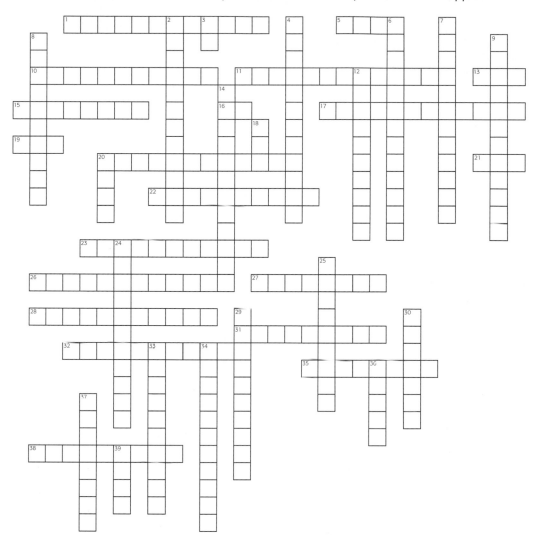

ACROSS

1. any syphilitic disease
5. same as pre- or before
10. inflammation of a uterine tube
11. condition of prolapsed uterus
13. hysterosalpingogram (abbrev.)
15. pertaining to a newborn
16. obstetrics (abbrev.)
17. painful, difficult menses
19. failure to thrive (abbrev.)
20. female disorders, physician specialist
21. prefix for eqal
22. incision into the abdominal wall
23. breast x-ray process
26. below the breast
27. pertaining to the neck of the uterus and the neck
28. using a scope to look into the abdomen
31. release of a matured ovum
32. never having a viable birth (adj.)
35. before birth (the fetus)
38. woman having many viable births

DOWN

2. pregnancy and delivery, physician specialist
3. pregnancy and delivery
4. abortion (abbrev.)
6. excision of only the uterus
7. condition of the uterine lining
8. menses (synonym)
9. excision of a breast instrument used to look into
12. the uterus
14. after delivery (the mother)
18. suture of the vaginal wall sexually transmitted infection (abbrev.)
20. pregnancy (abbrev.)
24. surgical repair of the breast
25. both sides
29. after intercourse
30. suffix for suture
33. after death
34. fixation of an ovary
36. prefix for unequal
37. same concentration as inside the cell
39. suffix for fixation

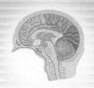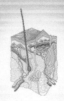

UNIT 8
Eye, Ear, Respiratory System, and Special Senses

Study these word parts, meanings, and examples. Then proceed to the first frame.

COMBINING FORMS

audi/o (hearing)
blephar/o (eyelid)
bronch/o (bronchus)
cor/e/o (pupil)
corne/o, kerat/o (cornea)
esthesi/o (feeling, sensation)
irid/o (iris)
kerat/o (cornea)
lacrim/o (tears)
laryng/o (larynx)
melan/o (black)
nas/o (nasal passage, nose)
nyct/o, noct/i (night)
ophthalm/o (eye)
opt/o (vision)
ot/o (ear)
phac/o (lens)
pharyng/o (pharynx)
phas/o (speech)
phon/o (sound)
phren/o (diaphragm)
pleur/o (pleural membrane)
pne/o (breathe)
pneum/o (air, lungs)
pneumon/o (lung)
presby/o (old)
pulmon/o (lung)
py/o (pus)
retin/o (retina)

rhin/o (nose)
scler/o (hard)
spir/o (respiration)
thorac/o (thorax)
trache/o (trachea)
tympan/o (eardrum)

PREFIXES

a/an– (lack of, without)
ambi– (both)
brady– (slow)
diplo– (double)
endo– (inner)
eso– (inward)
ex– (outside)
exo– (outward)
hypo– (below, down)
hyper– (above, upward)
my– (close)
tachy– (fast)
eu– (easy, good)
dys– (difficult, painful)

SUFFIXES

–algia (pain)
–eal (pertaining to)
–opia (vision)
–pnea (breathing)
–spasm (involuntary contraction)
–tropia (turning)

Word Examples

COMBING FORMS
audiometer
blepharedema
bronchoscope
corectasia
corneoplasty
anesthesia
iridoplegia
keratotomy
lacrimation
laryngitis
melanocyte
nasopharyngeal
nyctalopia
ophthalmic
optometrist
otorrhea
phacocele
pharyngoplasty
phasology
phonomyogram
phrenic
pleural
apnea
pneumothorax
pneumonia
presbyopia
pulmonary
pyogenic

retinoptosis
rhinoplasty
sclerectomy
respiratory
thoracocentesis
tracheostomy
tympanometry

PREFIXES
aphasia
ambiopia
bradypnea
diplopia
endotracheal
esotropia
exotropia
hyperopia
myopia
tachypnea
euphoria
dysphasia

SUFFIXES
blepharalgia
pharyngeal
presbyopia
orthopnea
blepharospasm
exotropia

ANSWER COLUMN

8-1

ot/o/rrhea
ō′ tō **rē′** ə

Ot/o/rrhea is both a sign and a disease. No matter which meaning is intended, discharge from the ear is _____.

8-2

ear
adjectival

Ot/o/rrhea means a discharging ear. **ot/o** is the combining form for _____. ot/ic is the _____ form.

8-3

-rrhea

The disease, otorrhea, involves discharge, inflammation, and deafness. One sign of this disease is found in its suffix, _____ , meaning discharge.

8-4

inflammation of
the ear

Otorrhea may be caused by ot/itis media. Ot/itis means
* _____.

8-5

ot/algia
ō **tal′** jē ə

Otitis media is common in children and usually causes **ear pain**. In medical terminology, ear pain is

_____.

8-6

otalgia

When ot/o/rrhea is prolonged, there has usually been enough destruction of the tissue that

_____ (ear pain) no longer occurs.

ANSWER COLUMN

ot/ic

ō′ tik

eardrum

tympan/o

8-7

Medication to be dropped into the ear is in a specially
prepared _____ (adjective) solution.

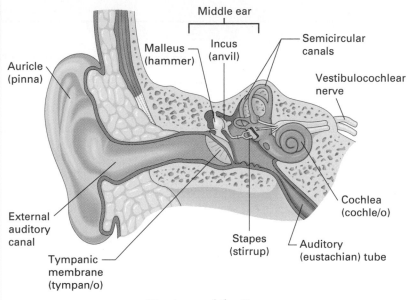

Middle ear

Malleus
(hammer)

Incus
(anvil)

Semicircular
canals

Vestibulocochlear
nerve

Auricle
(pinna)

External
auditory
canal

Tympanic
membrane
(tympan/o)

Stapes
(stirrup)

Cochlea
(cochle/o)

Auditory
(eustachian) tube

Structures of the Ear

8-8

Look up **tympanum** in your dictionary. The tympanum
is the _____. The combining form
for tympanum is _____.

ANSWER COLUMN

8-9

Build a word meaning:
pertaining to the eardrum (adjective)

tympan/ic, /al
tim **pan'** ik

_____ ;

incision into the eardrum

tympan/o/tomy
tim pan **ot'** ə mē

_____ ;

excision of the eardrum

tympan/ectomy
tim pan **ek'** tə mē

_____ .

NOTE: A common synonym for "tympanotomy" is "myringotomy."
myring/o is also a combining form for eardrum.

8-10

-meter is a suffix meaning instrument for measuring. The suffix
-metry indicates the process of measuring. The process of
measuring the function of the eardrum is

tympan/o/metry
tim pən **om'** et rē

called _____ .

Combining Form	Meaning	Suffixes
my/o	muscle	-graph (instrument for recording)
ech/o	reflected sound	-graphy (making a recording)
audi/o	hearing	-gram (record, picture)
phon/o	sound	-algia (pain)
phas/o	speech	-logy (study of)

ANSWER COLUMN

8-11

-phasia refers to conditions of speech. -phonia refers to conditions of sound or voice.

slow speech

Bradyphasia means *_____.

absence of voice

Aphonia means *_____.

pertaining to the voice

Phonic means *_____.

an instrument for
   measuring intensity
   of voice

A phonometer is *_____

_____.

8-12

phas/o means speech. Build the following terms related to speech.
unable to speak (without speech)

a/phasia
a **fā′** zē ə

_____;

slow speech

brady/phasia
brad i **fā′** zē ə

_____;

fast speech

tachy/phasia
tak i **fā′** zē ə

_____.

8-13

Build a term that means study of:
sound

phon/o/logy
fōn **ol′** o jē

_____;

hearing

audi/o/logy
aw dē **ol′** ō gē

_____;

speech

phas/o/logy
fā **zol′** ō jē

_____.

ANSWER COLUMN

8-14

audi/o is a combining form for hearing. The study of hearing is audi/o/logy. Build a term that means:
an instrument used to measure hearing

audi/o/meter
äw dē **om'** et er

_____ ;

the process of measuring hearing

audi/o/metry
äw dē **om'** et rē

_____ ;

a record made by the instrument used to test hearing

audi/o/gram
äw' dē ō gram

_____ .

8-15

Career Profile

Speech and language pathologists and audiologists assist physicians with diagnosis and treatment of language, speech, and hearing disorders. They may work in a hospital, school, clinic, or private office setting.

8-16

Recall that -rrhea is a suffix meaning flow or discharge. Rhinorrhea means discharge from the nose. **Rhin/o** is

nose
flow or discharge

used in words about the _____. -rrhea is
used to indicate *_____ .

8-17

Using what is necessary from **rhin/o**, form a word that means

rhin/itis
rī **nī'** tis

inflammation of the nose. _____ .

8-18

Rhin/o/rrhea is a symptom. Drainage from the nose due to upper respiratory infection (URI) is a symptom called

rhin/o/rrhea
rī nō **rē'** ə

_____ .

ANSWER COLUMN

---

rhin/o/plasty
rī′ nō plas tē

8-19

Nasal bone fractures may require surgery. Build a word that means surgical repair of the nose:

_____.

---

rhin/o/tomy
rī **not′** ə mē

8-20

Form a word that means incision of the nose:

_____.

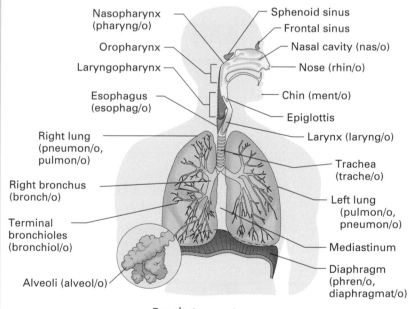

Nasopharynx (pharyng/o)

Oropharynx

Laryngopharynx

Esophagus (esophag/o)

Right lung (pneumon/o, pulmon/o)

Right bronchus (bronch/o)

Terminal bronchioles (bronchiol/o)

Alveoli (alveol/o)

Sphenoid sinus

Frontal sinus

Nasal cavity (nas/o)

Nose (rhin/o)

Chin (ment/o)

Epiglottis

Larynx (laryng/o)

Trachea (trache/o)

Left lung (pulmon/o, pneumon/o)

Mediastinum

Diaphragm (phren/o, diaphragmat/o)

Respiratory system

ANSWER COLUMN

8-21

Build a word meaning:
pertaining to the nose

nas/al
nā′ zəl

_____;

inflammation of the nose

nas/itis
nā **zī′** tis

_____;

instrument to examine the nose

nas/o/scope
nā′ zō skŏp

_____.

NOTE: You may also use "rhinitis" and "rhinoscope."

8-22

Build a word (you may use your dictionary if necessary) meaning:
inflammation of nose and pharynx

nas/o/pharyng/itis
nā′ zō far in **jī′** tis

_____;

pertaining to the nasal and frontal bones

nas/o/front/al
nā zō **fron′** təl

_____;

pertaining to the nose and lacrimal duct

nas/o/lacrim/al
nā zō **lak′** ri məl

_____.

8-23

The pharynx is the throat. Nas/o/pharyng/eal

nose and pharynx
(throat)

means pertaining to the *_____

_____.

8-24

pharynx (work on
the pronunciation)
fair′ inks

Pharyng/o is the combining form for pharynx. A Pharyng/o/myc/osis is a fungus disease of the

_____.

(Pronounced: fair ing′ ō mī **kō′** sis)

ANSWER COLUMN

8-25

Build a word meaning:
inflammation of the pharynx (throat)

pharyng/itis
fair in **jī′** tis

_____;

incision of the pharynx (throat)

pharyng/o/tomy
fair in **got′** ə mē

_____.

plural for pharynx;

pharyng/es
fair **in′** jēz

_____.

8-26

Build a word meaning (you put in diagonals):
disease of the throat

pharyng/o/pathy

_____;

surgical repair of the throat

pharyng/o/plasty

_____;

instrument to examine the throat

pharyng/o/scope

_____;

fungus condition of the throat

pharyng/o/myc/osis
(You pronounce)

_____.

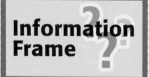

Information Frame

8-27

A sore throat, stuffy nose, and coughing are common complaints that may be symptoms of the common cold or respiratory seasonal allergies. However, some coughs are more severe, indicating an infection, asthma, emphysema, or even cancer. The table on the next page describes some common respiratory conditions related to coughing.

ANSWER COLUMN

8-28

Disease	Description
croup (kroōp)	Croup is a resonant barking cough caused by infection, allergy, or a foreign body, and occurs most often in children. Many types of respiratory congestion produce a croupy cough.
asthma (**az**′ mə)	Spasms of the bronchi cause a wheezing cough. This condition may be brought on by allergies, exercise, infection, or emotional stress.
emphysema (em fə **se**′ mə)	An overdistention of the air sacs (alveoli), caused by smoking tobacco, occurs due to loss of elasticity. Symptoms include: chronic cough, cyanosis, shortness of breath (SOB), and wheezing with long-term prognosis, often ending in respiratory and heart failure in severe cases.
pertussis (per **tus**′ is)	Also called whooping cough, this highly contagious infection is characterized by a cough with a shrill whooping inspiration. Most children are vaccinated against this infection with the DPT vaccine.

8-29

From what you have just learned, name the condition that matches the description below:

wheezing spastic cough

asthma

_____;

whooping cough

pertussis

_____;

difficulty breathing due to overdistention of the lungs from smoking

emphysema

_____.

8-30

laryng/o is used to build words that refer to the larynx (voice box). The larynx contains the vocal cords. When referring to the

larynx
lair′ inks
laryngo
(You pronounce)

_____ , use _____.

NOTE: **laryngo** is sometimes used to indicate "throat," as in otorhinolaryngologist (ENT).

ANSWER COLUMN

8-31

Form a word that means inflammation of the larynx
(voice box): _____.

laryng/itis
lair' in **jī'** tis

8-32

After a bad cold, a patient may have laryngitis with accompanying
pain. Pain in the voice box is called

_____.

laryng/algia
lair' in **gal'** jē ə

8-33

Anything that obstructs the flow of air from the nose to the larynx
may call for creating a new opening, or a

_____.

laryng/ostomy
lair' in **gos'** tō mē

8-34

When a **temporary opening** in the voice box is made, the surgical
procedure is a laryng/**o/tomy**. An incision into the larynx is called a

_____.

laryng/o/tomy
lair' in **got'** ə mē

8-35

Build a word meaning:
any disease of the voice box

_____;

laryng/o/pathy
lair in **gop'** ə thē

instrument used to examine the voice box

_____;

laryng/o/scope
lair **in'** gō skōp

spasm of the voice box

_____;

laryng/o/spasm
lair **in'** gō spazm

singular of larynges

_____;

larynx
lair' inks

ANSWER COLUMN

8-36

Py/osis is a condition with pus formation.
Trache/o/py/osis means *_____

a condition of the
   trachea with
   pus formation

_____.

8-37

hemorrhage from
   the trachea (windpipe)

Trache/o/rrhagia means *_____

_____.

8-38

Build a word meaning:
pain in the windpipe

trache/algia
trā kē **al′** jē ə

_____;

incision into the windpipe

trache/o/tomy
trā kē **ot′** ə mē

_____.

8-39

Build a word meaning:
examination of the trachea

trache/o/scopy
trā′ kē **os′** kō pē

_____;

pertaining to the trachea

trache/al
trā′ kē əl

_____;

incision of trachea and larynx

trache/o/laryng/o/tomy
trā′ kē ō lair in **got′** ə mē

_____;

form a new opening in the trachea

trache/o/stomy
trā′ kē **os′** tə mē

_____;

within the trachea

endo/trache/al
en dō **trā′** kē əl

_____.

ANSWER COLUMN

8-40

inflammation of
   the bronchi

Bronch/itis means *_____
_____.

an instrument to
   examine the
   bronchi

A bronch/o/scope is *_____
_____.

8-41

Build a word meaning:
calculus in a bronchus

bronch/o/lith
bron' kō lith

_____ ;

examination of a bronchus (with instrument)

bronch/o/scopy
bron **kos'** kō pē

_____ ;

bronch/o/rrhagia
bron kō **rā'** jē ə

bronchial hemorrhage

_____ ;

plural of bronchus

bronch/i
bron kī

_____.

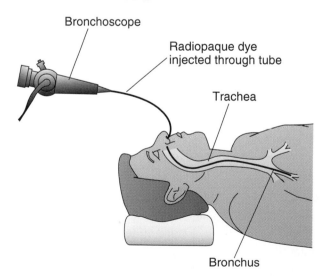

Bronchoscope

Radiopaque dye
injected through tube

Trachea

Bronchus

Fiberoptic bronchoscopy

ANSWER COLUMN

	8-42
	Build a word meaning:
	formation of a new opening into a bronchus
bronch/o/stomy	_____;
	spasm of a bronchus
bronch/o/spasm	_____;
	suturing of a bronchus
bronch/o/rrhaphy	_____.
(You pronounce)	
	8-43
	Pleur/al means
pertaining to the	* _____.
pleura	
	Pleur/itis means
inflammation of	* _____.
the pleura	
	8-44
	Build a word meaning:
	pain in the pleura
pleur/algia	_____;
plōō **ral'** jē ə	
	surgical puncturing of the pleura
pleur/o/centesis	_____.
plōō rō sen **tē'** sis	

Information Frame ??

8-45

Look up the word "pleurisy." Read all your dictionary has to say about this disease. A synonym is pleuritis.

ANSWER COLUMN

8-46

Inflammation of the pleura is pleuritis, or

pleur/isy
plo͞o′ ri sē

_____.

8-47

phren/o refers to the diaphragm, which is the muscle located below the lungs. The phren/ic nerve innervates

diaphragm
dī′ ə fram
(silent g)

the _____.

8-48

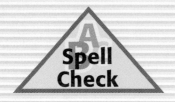
Spell Check

Watch the silent "g" in diaphragm. Look this word up in your dictionary and you will find there are several different types of diaphragms. In the respiratory system, the diaphragmatic muscle is the major inspiratory muscle. Remember, don't say the "g," but do spell with the "g."

8-49

Build a word meaning:
pain in the diaphragm

phren/algia
fren **al′** jē ə

_____;

pertaining to the diaphragm and the stomach

phren/o/gastr/ic
fren ō **gas′** trik

_____.

8-50

pne/o comes from the Greek word "pneuma," breathing.
pne/o used anyplace in a word means

breathe or
breathing

* _____.

ANSWER COLUMN

8-51

Review the **"p" rule** on the inside front cover. When pne/o begins a word, the "p" is silent. When **pne/o** occurs later in a word, the "p" is pronounced. In tachypnea, the

pronounced

"p" is _____.

8-52

slow breathing
tachy/pnea
ta **kip'** nē ə

brady- is a prefix for slow. Brady/pnea means

* _____. A word for rapid

breathing is _____.

8-53

tachy- is a prefix for fast. The rate of respiration (breathing) is controlled by the amount of carbon dioxide in the blood. Increased carbon dioxide speeds up breathing and causes

tachypnea
ta **kip'** nē ə

_____.

8-54

Muscle exercise increases the amount of carbon dioxide in the blood. This speeds respiration and produces

tachypnea

_____.

8-55

tachypnea

Running a race causes _____.

8-56

a- is a prefix meaning without. **A**/pnea literally means

without breathing

* _____.

ANSWER COLUMN

8-57

Apnea means cessation of breathing for more than 20 seconds.
If the level of carbon dioxide in the blood falls very low,

a/pnea
ap' nē ə
_____ results.

8-58

apnea
When breathing ceases for a bit, _____
results. If breathing is merely very slow, it is called

brady/pnea
brad' **ip'** nē ə
_____.

8-59

bad, painful, or
 difficult
well or easy
dys- means *_____.
The opposite of dys is eu. eu means
*_____.

8-60

Form the word that means the opposite of:
dys/pnea

eu/pnea
yo͞op **nē'** ə
eu/phoria
yo͞o **for' ē** ə
_____;

dys/phoria

_____.

Notice how these word roots were built from each other.

Combining Form	Meaning	Medical Term
pne/o	breathing	tachy**pnea**
pneum/o	air	**pne**umothorax
pneumon/o	lung	**pne**umonectomy

ANSWER COLUMN

8-61

The lungs are the organs of the body that take in air (breathe). **Pne**umon/o is used in medical words concerning lungs.

Pneumon/ectomy means

excision of a lung

*_____.

Incision of a lung is a

pneumon/o/tomy
noo' mə **nô'** tə mē

_____.

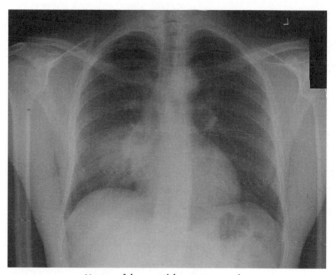

X-ray of lung with pneumonia

8-62

any disease of
the lungs

Pneumon/o/pathy means

*_____.

Form a word meaning hemorrhage of a lung.

pneumon/o/rrhagia
noo' mə nō **rā'** jē ə

_____

ANSWER COLUMN

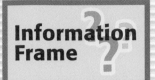

8-63

Pneumonia is an acute inflammation in a generalized diffuse area of the lungs caused by a variety of organisms and viruses. Antibiotics are used most to treat bacterial pneumonia. Another word for pneumonia is pneumonitis. **Pneumonitis** is usually used when a localized area of inflammation of the lung occurs.

8-64

Recall that -centesis means surgical puncture.
Form a word meaning surgical puncture of a lung.

pneumon/o/centesis
nōō′ mə nō sen **tē′** sis

_____.

8-65

Two words meaning inflammation of the lungs are:

pneumon/ia
nōō′ **mōn′** ya
pneumon/itis
nōō′ mə **nī′** tis

_____

and

_____.

8-66

Lung tissue that has detached from the chest wall may be surgically reattached (fixated) by a procedure called:

pneumon/o/pexy
nōō′ mə nō pek′ sē

_____.

8-67

Pneumon/o/melan/osis is a lung disease in which lung tissue becomes black due to breathing black dust. The word

melan

root for black is _____.

ANSWER COLUMN

8-68

Pneumon/o/melan/osis literally means a condition of black lungs. Analyze this word.

pneumon/o

melan

osis

_____ combining form for lung

_____ word root for black

_____ suffix—condition

8-69

The inhalation (breathing) of black dust results in

pneumonomelanosis

nōō′ mə nō mel ə **nō′** sis

pneumonomelanosis

_____.

The inhalation of much soot or black smoke can also

cause _____.

8-70

Information Frame ??

Pneum/o and **pneumon/o** can both refer to the lung. **Pneum/o** is derived from the Greek word "pneuma" (for air). **Pneum/o** is used in words to mean air.

8-71

pneumon/o comes from the Greek word "pneumon" (lung). **pneumon/o** is used in words that refer to the

lung or lungs

*_____.

8-72

air

pneum/o is used in most words to mean _____, as in pneumatic drill, but it can also mean lung.

8-73

Your use of **pneum/o** will be in words about air or lung. Pneum/o/derm/a means a collection of air under the skin. A collection of air in the chest cavity (thorax)

pneum/o/thorax

nōō mō **thôr′** aks

is a _____.

ANSWER COLUMN

8-74

The combining form for thorax (chest cavity) is

thorac/o

_____. The adjective that
pertains to a collection of air in the chest cavity is

pneum/o/thorac/ic
(You pronounce)

_____.

8-75

A tach/o/meter in cars measures the number of revolutions per
minute of the drive shaft. An instrument that measures air volume in
respiration is a

pneum/o/meter
nōō **mom'** et er

_____.

8-76

A collection of air and serum in the chest cavity is
pneum/o/ser/o/thorax. A collection of air and pus in the thoracic
cavity is a

pneum/o/py/o/thorax

_____,
while a collection of air and blood in this same cavity

pneum/o/hem/o/thorax
(You pronounce)

is a _____.

8-77

Pulmonary and pulmonic are both used as adjectives meaning
pertaining to the lungs. **pulmon/o** is another combining form for
lung used only in a few words. The heart valve through which
blood travels to the lungs is the

pulmon/ary
pul' mō nair ē

_____ valve.

8-78

Blood flows from the heart to the lungs via the

pulmon/ary or
pulmon/ic
pul **mon'** ik

_____ artery.

ANSWER COLUMN

8-79

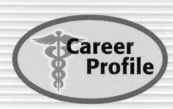

Career Profile

Respiratory therapists and respiratory therapy technicians administer oxygen and various types of gases or aerosol drugs for treatment of lung and heart disease. They also perform respiratory function tests.

8-80

Information Frame

Right and left. Eyes and ears. It is important when describing symptoms to note the correct structures. Because eyes, ears, and tympanic membranes have right and left structures, they are often designated by the following abbreviations:

OD	oculus dexter (eye, right)
OS	oculus sinister (eye, left)
AD	auris dextra (ear, right)
AS	auris sinistra (ear, left)
MTD	membrana tympani dexter (eardrum, right)
MTS	membrana tympani sinister (eardrum, left)

8-81

inflammation of the eye
pertaining to the eye

ophthalm/o is used in words to mean eye. Ophthalm/itis means *_____.
Ophthalm/ic means *_____.

8-82

pain in the eye

Ophthalm/algia means
*_____.

8-83

Spell Check

Before building words with **ophthalm/o**, be sure you have the **phth** order of o**phth**alm/o straight. Pronounce it **off thalm' ō**, *not* op **tal'** mō.

ANSWER COLUMN

	8-84
	Build a word meaning:
	herniation of an eye (abnormal protrusion)
ophthalm/o/cele	_____;
of **thal'** mō sēl	
	instrument for measuring the eye
ophthalm/o/meter	_____.
of' thal **mom'** ə ter	

	8-85
	Build a word meaning:
	any eye disease
ophthalm/o/pathy	_____;
	plastic surgery of the eye
ophthalm/o/plasty	_____.
(You pronounce)	

	8-86
	Ophthalm/o/logy is the medical specialty dealing with eye disease. We call the physician who practices this specialty an
ophthalm/o/logist	_____.
of' thal **mol'** ō jist	

	8-87
	Ophthalm/o/scopy is the examination of the interior of the eye. The instrument used for this examination is an
ophthalm/o/scope	_____.
of thal' mō skōp	

The table below analyzes word parts pertaining to the eye and vision:

Word/Part	Use
-op/ia	suffix for vision
opt/ic	adjective—pertaining to vision
opt/o	combining form for vision or eye
ophthalm/o	combining form for eye

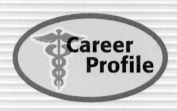

Career Profile

8-88

Optometrists (OD) and optometric assistants (COA) and technicians (COT): Optometrists measure visual acuity, prescribe corrective lenses as needed, and examine the eye for disease. Assistants and technicians assist with exams, perform tests, prepare corrective lenses for dispensing, and teach patients.

8-89

Build a word meaning:
one who measures visual acuity

_____ ;

opt/o/metrist
op **to'** met rist

the cranial nerve for vision (adjective)

_____ ;

opt/ic
op' tik

the measurement of vision

_____ .

opt/o/metry
op **to'** me trē

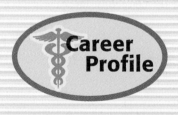

Career Profile

8-90

Notice the difference between the following:
Ophthalm/o/logist—physician (MD or DO) specializing in treating diseases of the eye with medication and surgery.
Opt/o/metr/ist—licensed practitioner (OD—optometric doctor) limited to eye examinations and prescribing corrective lenses. Both are called doctor.

ANSWER COLUMN

8-91

-opia is used as a suffix to denote a condition of vision. Look up the following terms and note the type of vision they are describing:

nearsightedness   myopia   * _____ ;

farsightedness   hyperopia   * _____ ;

loss of accommodation   presbyopia   * _____ ;
   (old eye)

double vision   diplopia   * _____ .

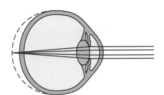

Hyperopia
(farsightedness)
Light rays focus behind the retina

Far objects focus better on the retina than close objects.

8-92

my/opia   If you can see near objects well but have difficulty with faraway

mi **o′** pē ə   objects, you may have _____ .

hyper/opia   If you can see far away better than near to you, you may have

hī per **ō′** pē ə   _____ .

8-93

    Blephar/o/ptosis means prolapse of an eyelid.

blephar/o   The combining form for eyelid is _____ .

8-94

    "Blepharedema" means swelling of the

eyelid   _____ .

    blephar/o makes you think of the

eyelid   _____ .

ANSWER COLUMN

8-95

Blephar/edema means swelling or puffiness of the eyelid. Build a word that means:
inflammation of an eyelid

blephar/itis
blef ə **rī'** tis

_____;

incision of an eyelid

blephar/otomy
blef ə **rot'** ə mē

_____.

8-96

Another combining form for eyelid is **palpebr/o**. To palpebrate is to wink. Palpebr/itis would mean the same

blephar/itis

as _____.

8-97

Look up "cornea" in your dictionary. Look at the words in your dictionary that begin with **corne**. A combining form for **cornea**

corne/o

is _____.

8-98

While thinking of the meaning, analyze:
corneitis

corne/itis
kôr' nē **ī'** tis

_____;

corneoiritis

corne/o/ir/itis
kôr' nē ō ī **rī'** tis

_____;

corneoscleral

corne/o/scler/al
kôr' nē ō **skler'** əl

_____.

ANSWER COLUMN

ir
scler

8-99

From the preceding frame, find two other word roots that match labels on your drawing. They are _____ and _____.

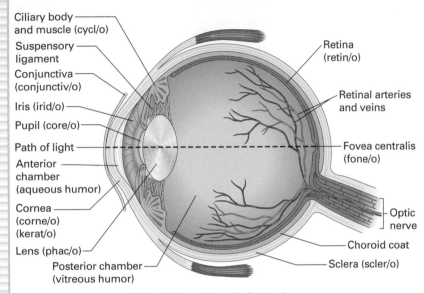

Ciliary body
and muscle (cycl/o)
Suspensory
ligament
Conjunctiva
(conjunctiv/o)
Iris (irid/o)
Pupil (core/o)
Path of light
Anterior
chamber
(aqueous humor)
Cornea
(corne/o)
(kerat/o)
Lens (phac/o)
Posterior chamber
(vitreous humor)

Retina
(retin/o)
Retinal arteries
and veins
Fovea centralis
(fone/o)
Optic
nerve
Choroid coat
Sclera (scler/o)

Lateral view of eyeball interior

8-100

phac/o/cele
fā′ kō sēl

phac/o is the combining form for the lens of the eye. Build a word that means herniation or displacement of the lens

_____.

8-101

phac/o/emulsification
fā′ kō ēm ul si fi **kā′** shən

Cataracts may be treated with an ultrasonic device to emulsify the lens for removal. This procedure is called

_____ emulsification.

ANSWER COLUMN

sclera
skler′ ə

8-102

Look up the first word in your dictionary beginning with scler. It is _____.

8-103

Read what the sclera is. Does the word root plus the meaning of the Greek word from which it is derived suggest an already familiar combining form to you?

scler/o
hard

It is _____, which means _____.

8-104

The sclera of the eye is the "hard" outer coat of the eye.
Build a word meaning:
pertaining to the sclera (adjective)

scler/al
skler′ əl

_____;

excision of the sclera (or part)

scler/ectomy
skle **rek′** tə mē

_____;

formation of an opening into the sclera

scler/ostomy
skler **os′** tə mē

_____.

8-105

Go back to the other word root you found in **Frame 8-99**. With it in mind, find the part of the eye (on the illustration on page 308) to which it refers. This is the

iris
ī′ ris

_____.

ANSWER COLUMN

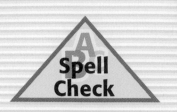

8-106

Look up "iris" in your dictionary. **ir** is one word root for the iris. It is limited in use. It is always used to express inflammation, so you can see it is important if limited in use, as in "iritis."

8-107

With the information in **Frame 8-106** and the word root you found, build a word meaning:

inflammation of the iris

ir/itis

_____ ;

inflammation of the cornea and iris

corne/o/ir/itis

_____ ;

inflammation of the sclera and iris

scler/o/ir/itis
(You pronounce)

_____ .

8-108

In your dictionary, find the plural of **iris**. It is

ir/ides
ir′ i dēz, **ī′** ri dēz

_____ .

8-109

With your dictionary, find the combining form for "iris." It

irid/o

is _____ .

ANSWER COLUMN

8-110

Using the combining form for "irid," build a word meaning:
herniation of the iris

irid/o/cele
ī **rid′** ō sel

_____;

pain in the iris

irid/algia
ī ri **dal′** jē ə

_____;

excision of part of the iris

irid/ectomy
ī ri **dek′** tə mē

_____.

8-111

The following forms make you think of:

iris   ir _____;

iris   irid/o _____;

sclera (hard)   scler/o _____;

cornea   corne/o _____.

8-112

Look up **retina** in your dictionary. Read about the retina. Look at the words beginning with **retin** in your dictionary. The combining form for words about the retina is _____.

retin/o

8-113

Build a word meaning:
pertaining to the retina

retin/al
ret′ in əl

_____;

inflammation of the retina

retin/itis
ret in **ī′** tis

_____;

repair of a detached retina

retin/o/plasty
ret′ i nō plas tē

_____.

ANSWER COLUMN

8-114

The instrument used to examine the retina is the

_____.

retin/o/scope
ret' in ō skōp
retin/o/scopy
ret' in **os'** ko pē

The process of examining the retina is

_____.

8-115

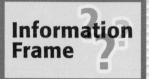

Information Frame

The pupil in the eye is the opening in the iris through which light passes. Identify the pupil in the illustration of the eye on page 308. The word root for pupil is **cor** or **core**.

8-116

The combining form for pupil is **cor/e/o**. Build a word meaning:
pupil misplaced

cor/ectopia
kôr ek **tō'** pē ə

_____ /ectopia _____;

destruction of the pupil

cor/e/lysis
kôr **el'** ə sis

_____ /lysis _____;

dilatation (stretching) of the pupil

cor/ectasia (is)
kôr ek **tā'** zhə

_____ /ectasia _____;

unequal pupil size

anis/o/coria
an ī sō **kôr'** ē ə

_____.

ANSWER COLUMN

8-117

core/o is also used as a combining form for pupil. Using **core/o**, build a word meaning:

instrument for measuring the pupil

core/o/meter

_____;

measurement of the pupil

core/o/metry

_____;

plastic surgery of the pupil

core/o/plasty
(You pronounce)

_____.

8-118

cor

Whether **cor/e** or **cor/o** is used, the word root for "pupil of the eye" is _____.

8-119

corne

You have already learned one word root for cornea. It is _____. Another word root for "cornea" is **kerat**, and it is the more commonly used form.

8-120

The word root most commonly used for cornea is

kerat
kerat/o

_____. The combining form is

_____.

8-121

Using kerat/o build a word meaning:

herniation of the cornea

kerat/o/cele
ker′ ə tō sēl

_____;

plastic operation of the cornea (corneal transplant)

kerat/o/plasty
ker′ ə tō plas′ tē

_____.

ANSWER COLUMN

8-122

Build a word meaning:
incision of the cornea

kerat/o/tomy

_____;

inflammation of cornea and sclera

kerat/o/scler/itis
(You pronounce)

_____.

8-123

The following forms make you think of:

retina   retin/o _____;
pupil   cor/e _____;
pupil   core/o _____;
cornea   kerat/o _____.

8-124

Look up lacrim/al in your dictionary. Lacrimal is a word
that means pertaining to _____.

tears

8-125

The gland that secretes tears is the

lacrim/al
lak' ri məl

_____ gland.

8-126

The sac that collects lacrimal fluid is the

lacrimal

_____ sac.

8-127

Lacrimal fluid is drained away by means of the

nas/o/lacrim/al
nā zō **lak'** ri məl

 nas o _____duct.

ANSWER COLUMN

8-128

Lacrimal fluid keeps the surface of the eye moistened. It is continually forming and being removed. When there is more formed than can be removed by the apparatus, you say the person is

crying or tearing   * _____.

8-129

If you can see close objects but not distant ones, you may have my/opia, or "close vision." Presby/opia is experienced by older people as a loss of accommodation by the lens. The word means "old vision." In each of these terms, the suffix for vision is

opia   _____.

8-130

amb/i means both or both sides. Amb/i/later/al means

both   pertaining to _____ sides.

8-131

An amb/i/dextr/ous person can work well with

both   _____ hands.

8-132

A word that means both eyes form separate images

amb/i/opia   (vision) is _____.
am bē ō′ pē ə

8-133

The result of separate vision from both eyes is a double image or double vision. Medically, double vision can be expressed either

dipl/opia   as _____ or
amb/i/opia   _____.

ANSWER COLUMN

8-134

Hyper/opia means farsightedness (able to focus on objects at a distance). The opposite of hyperopia is nearsightedness

my/opia
mī ō′ pē ə

or _____.

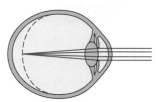

Myopia
(nearsightedness)
Light rays focus in front of the retina

Myopia (nearsightedness)

8-135

Recall that **nyct/o** means night. **al** is a word root meaning not. Nyct/al/opia means unable to see at night and has several causes. Retinal fatigue from exposure to very bright light is a cause of

nyctalopia
nik al ō′ pē ə

_____.

8-136

Retinitis pigmentosa is another cause of

nyctalopia

_____.

ANSWER COLUMN

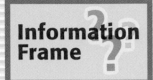

Information Frame

8-137

"*Strabismos*" is a Greek word meaning squinting. From this the medical term "strabismus," also called squint, is used to indicate an abnormal movement or direction of the eye (visual axis) inward, outward, upward, or down that cannot be controlled by the person. Strabismus, or squinting, may occur in one eye or both and is treated by surgery. "*Trope*," another Greek word, means turning, and the suffix -tropia is used to build words related to the turning or position of the eye. All of the following conditions are a specific type of strabismus:

Condition	Description
exo/tropia	eyes (visual axis) pointing outward (external)
eso/tropia	eyes (visual axis) pointing inward (convergent)
hyper/tropia	eyes (visual axis) pointing upward
hypo/tropia	eyes (visual axis) pointing downward

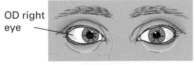

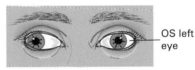

OD right eye   OS left eye

(A) Esotropia   **(B) Exotropia**

8-138

Look up "strabismus" in your medical dictionary and you may find that there are over 20 types of strabismus.

8-139

The term used to indicate an inward convergence of the eyes (cross-eyed) is called _____.

eso/tropia
es ō **tro'** pē ə

ANSWER COLUMN

8-140

Build a word that means a condition in which the muscle bears the eye in an upward position: _____.

hyper/tropia
hī per **trō'** pē ə

8-141

An abnormal condition that effects the position of the eye's axis and focus either up, down, out, or in is called _____.

strabismus
str ə **biz'** məs

8-142

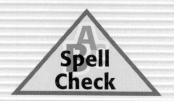

Here's a word you do not want to confuse with strabismus—it is "**astigmatism**." Astigmatism (a- meaning not, **stigma**, meaning point) is caused by an unequal curvature of the surface of the eye diffusing the focal point on the retina. It is treated using corrective lenses. Most general vision exams screen for astigmatism.

a/stigma/tism
ə **stig'** mə tizm

8-143

A condition causing a blurring or twinkling sensation when distant points of light are viewed and focused with corrective lenses is _____.

a/stigma/tism

8-144

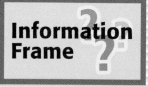

"Esthesia" is a word meaning physical feeling or sensation. an- is a form of the prefix a-, an- means without (i.e., anemia, anorexia).

ANSWER COLUMN

Spell Check

an/esthesia
an es **thēs'** ē ə

an/esthesi/o/logy
an es thes ē **ol'** o jē

an/esthet/ist
an **es'** the tist

8-145

Watch out for the letter change when using esthesi/o. The "s" changes to "t" in anesthe**t**ist and anesthe**t**ic.
Use your medical dictionary to analyze the following words by dividing them into their word parts:
anesthesia

_____;

anesthesiology

_____;

anesthetist

_____.

anesthe/tic
an es **the'** tik

8-146

Novocaine is used to remove sensation in a specified area.
It is a local _____.

oversensitivity to pain
or hyperesthesia

8-147

Algesia is a noun meaning oversensitivity to pain. Hyper/esthesi/a is a synonym for algesia. "Algesia" means

_____.

8-148

Use the word root **alges** to build a word meaning:
instrument used to measure pain

alges/i/meter
al **jē′ se′** met er

_____;

pertaining to pain (adjective)

alges/ic
al **jē′** sik

_____;

condition without pain (noun)

an/alges/ia
an al **jē′** sē ə

_____;

pertaining to antipain medication (adjective)

an/alges/ic
an al **jē** siḱ

_____.

8-149

a- and an- are prefixes that mean without. Examine the following list of words.

a-	an-
a/bi/o/tic	an/al/gesia
a/blast/emic	an/aphy/laxis
a/cholia	an/emia
a/derma	an/encephalus
a/febrile	an/esthesia
a/galactia	an/iso/cyt/osis
a/kinesia	an/hidr/osis
a/lalia	an/iridia
a/men/o/rrhea	an/onychia
a/pnea	an/orexia
a/reflexia	an/uria
a/sepsis	an/uresis

ANSWER COLUMN

8-150

Draw a conclusion.

Use a- if it is followed by a (vowel-consonant)

consonant

_____.

Use an- if it is followed by a (vowel/consonant)

vowel

_____.

The following medical abbreviations correspond to the terms in Unit 8.

ABBREVIATION	MEANING
AD	right ear (auris dextra)
AS	left ear (auris sinistra)
CCC-A	Certificate of Clinical Competency in Audiology
COPD	chronic obstructive pulmonary disease
ENT	ear, nose, and throat (specialist)
HEENT	head, eyes, ears, nose, throat
L+A	light and accommodation
MTD	right eardrum (membrana tympani dexter)
MTS	left eardrum (membrana tympani sinister)
OD	right eye (oculus dexter)
OM	otitis media
OS, OL	left eye (oculus sinister, oculus laevus)
OU	both eyes (oculus uterque)
PERRLA	pupils equal, round, reactive to light, and accommodation
SOB	shortness of breath
TB, Tb	tuberculosis
URI	upper respiratory infection

You have been introduced to many new terms in this unit. To make sure you know them well, work the review exercises on the following pages. Also, listen to the CD-ROM accompanying the third edition of *Medical Terminology Made Easy* and practice pronunciation.

**UNIT 8
REVIEW EXERCISES**

Part 1: Review the terms you have learned in this unit by drawing the diagonal lines between the word parts and writing the meaning of each term. Use your medical dictionary or the frames if you need help. After you have completed these tasks, say each term aloud to practice pronunciation.

1. ambiopia _____

2. analgesia _____

3. anesthesiology _____

4. aphasia _____

5. aphonia _____

6. atelectasis _____

7. audiology _____

8. audiometer _____

9. blepharedema _____

10. bradypnea _____

11. bronchospasm _____

12. corectasia _____

13. corneoiritis _____

14. croup _____

15. dyspnea _____

16. emphysema _____

17. exotropia _____

18. hypertropia _____

19. iridocele _____

20. keratotomy _____

21. laryngitis _____

22. laryngoscopy _____

23. myopia _____

24. nasolacrimal _____

25. nasopharyngitis _____

26. nyctalopia _____

27. ophthalmologist _____

UNIT 8
REVIEW EXERCISES

28. ophthalmometer   _____

29. ophthalmoscope   _____

30. optometrist   _____

31. otalgia   _____

32. otorrhea   _____

33. phacoemulsification   _____

34. pharyngomycosis   _____

35. pleurocentesis   _____

36. pneumonomelanosis   _____

37. pneumonorrhagia   _____

38. pneumothorax   _____

39. presbyopia   _____

40. pulmonary   _____

41. retinopexy   _____

42. rhinolith   _____

43. rhinoplasty   _____

44. sclerectomy   _____

45. strabismus   _____

46. tracheostomy   _____

47. tachyphasia   _____

48. tachypnea   _____

49. tympanotomy   _____

Part 2: Write the medical term that means:

1. incision into the eardrum _____

2. inflammation of the nose and pharynx _____

3. inability to speak _____

4. instrument used to measure hearing _____

5. flow of tears _____

6. poor vision at night _____

7. herniation of the iris _____

UNIT 8
REVIEW EXERCISES

8. inflammation of the eyelid _____

9. instrument used to examine the eyes _____

10. farsightedness _____

Part 3: Match each term with its correct meaning.

_____ 1. otorrhea	a. removal of part of the diaphragm
_____ 2. laryngostomy	b. excision of the diaphragm
_____ 3. pneumonia	c. inflammation of the voice box
_____ 4. pneumothorax	d. physician specializing in eye diseases
_____ 5. audiometry	e. difficulty hearing
_____ 6. tachypnea	f. unable to make a sound
_____ 7. aphasia	g. unable to speak
_____ 8. bronchorrhagia	h. lack of breathing
_____ 9. phrenectomy	i. measurement of hearing
_____ 10. optometry	j. abnormally fast breathing
	k. air in the chest cavity
	l. flow or discharge from the ear
	m. hemorrhage of the bronchi
	n. specialty in vision measurement
	o. slow heart rate
	p. flow or discharge from the foot
	q. pneumonitis
	r. form a new opening in the voice box

UNIT 8
REVIEW EXERCISES

Part 4: Use the medical terms listed below to complete these sentences:

myopia	otalgia	otic	tympanotomy
audiologist	rhinorrhea	rhinoplasty	pharyngoscope
nasolacrimal	laryngectomy	endotracheal	bronchorrhagia
diaphragm	pleurisy	pneumonia	tachypnea
bradypnea	apnea	pneumothorax	pulmonary
aphonia	aphasia	keratotomy	anisocoria
nyctalopia			

1. Mrs. Thom Katz is quite upset because she has difficulty seeing at night. Her doctor says her diagnosis is:

2. You may use a (an) _____ as a contraceptive, and you use your _____ to breathe.

3. Swelling and fluid buildup in the lung tissue is _____ edema.

4. Mr. Vic Tims was stabbed in the chest, allowing air to enter the chest cavity. This caused a _____ and the lung to collapse. He was also hit in the head and suffered a concussion. When his pupils were checked, he had

   _____.

5. The _____ said that Joe's hearing was within normal limits. But the optometrist found he could only see objects close to himself. Dx: _____. A surgical option to wear glasses, called "radial _____," was discussed with an ophthalmologist.

6. After her stroke, Harriet experienced _____ and could not seem to match the correct words with what she wanted to say.

7. To assist the drowning victim's breathing by keeping the airway open, a (an) _____ tube was inserted and CPR continued until the patient revived.

UNIT 8
REVIEW EXERCISES

Part 5: Draw a line to match the abbreviation with its meaning.

1. L+A

2. OD

3. AS

4. TB

5. OS

6. ENT

7. COPD

8. URI

tuberculosis

right eye

optometrist

chronic obstructive pulmonary disease

upper respiratory infection

ophthalmologist

otorhinolaryngologist

left ear

light and accommodation

left eye

**UNIT 8
REVIEW EXERCISES**

Part 6: Label the structures of the eye. Then draw a line to the combining form that matches that structure.

1. corne/o   _____

2. retin/o   _____

3. scler/o   _____

4. cycl/o   _____

5. core/o   _____

6. phac/o   _____

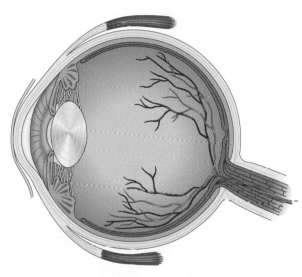

Lateral view of eyeball interior

Unit 8 Puzzle

As a self-test work the crossword puzzle and then check your answers in Appendix F.

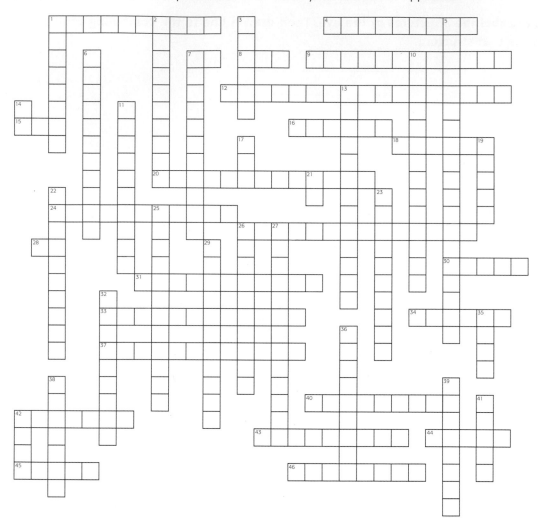

ACROSS

1. old eye (vision)
4. used to look into the nose
7. left eye (abbrev.)
8. upper respiratory infection
9. surgical repair of the retina
12. black lung disease (condition)
15. prefix for difficult or painful
16. disease with wheezing, spasms of the bronchi
18. combining form for air
20. pertaining to the cornea and sclera
24. nose job
26. hemorrhage of the bronchi
28. right ear
30. combining form for hearing
31. same as pneumonia
33. within the trachea
34. noun for chest
37. new opening in the trachea for breathing
40. cross-eyed
42. ear pain
43. difficulty making sounds with the voice
44. suffix for flow or discharge
45. absence of breathing
46. plural of larynx

DOWN

1. same as pleuritis
2. pertaining to the eye
3. strabismus
5. destruction of the lens for removal
6. inflammation of the eyelid
7. vision specialist
10. surgical repair of the throat
11. night blindness
13. protrusion (herniation) of the eye
14. optometric doctor (abbrev.)
17. combining form for ear
19. pertaining to vision
21. prefix for easy or good
22. excision of the iris
23. incision into the cornea
25. used to look at the voice box
26. inflammation of the bronchi
27. practice or study of eye diseases
29. incision into the eardrum
32. whooping cough
35. prefix for both
36. study of hearing
38. singular for pharynges
39. pertaining to the tear ducts
41. head, eye, ear, nose, and throat (abbrev.)
42. suffix for vision

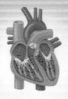

UNIT 9
Directions and Regions of the Body

You will use the following word parts to build terms about directions and regions of the body in this unit. Study these word parts, meanings, and examples. Then proceed to the first frame.

COMBINING FORMS

chir/o (hand)
cost/o (rib)
crani/o (skull)
dextr/o (right)
fus/o (melting, flowing)
gastr/o (stomach)
later/o (side)
lumb/o (lumbar spine)
pod/o, ped/i (foot)
pub/o (pubis)
sinistr/o (left)
son/o (sound)
ven/o (vein)
vers/ion (turning, twisting)

PREFIXES

ab- (away from)
ad- (toward)
ante- (front, before)
circum- (encircling, around)
con- (with)
contra- (against)
dia- (through)
dis- (to free of, separate, or undo)
epi- (upon, on top of)
extra- (outside of)
hemi- (half)

hetero- (different)
homo- (same)
in- (into, not)
infra- (below)
intra- (within)
macro- (large)
meta- (beyond)
micro- (small)
para- (abnormal, near, beyond)
per- (through)
peri- (around or near)
retro- (behind)
semi- (half)
sub- (under, below)
super- (above, over)
supra- (above, over)
trans- (across)
ultra- (beyond, in excess)

SUFFIXES

-ia (condition)
-ia, ar, ic, al, ac, ous (adjective endings pertaining to, relating to)
-graphy (process of making a picture)
-iatric (pertaining to a specialty)
-stasis (controlling, stopping)
-plasty (surgical repair)
-tion, sion, ia, us, ive (noun endings)

Word Examples

COMBINING FORMS
chiropractor
intercostal
intracranial
dextral
infusion
hypogastric
bilateral
supralumbar
podiatry
suprapubic
sinistral
sonography
intravenous
anteversion

PREFIXES
abduction
adhesion
anteflexion
circumscribed
congenital
contraindicated
diathermy
disassociate
epidural
extra-articular
hemigastrectomy
heterosexual

homolateral
incontinence
inframammary
intramuscular
macrodactylia
metacarpals
microcardia
paraplegia
percutaneous
pericardium
retrosternal
semiconscious
subglossal
superinfection
supracranial
transposition
ultraviolet

SUFFIXES
hemiplegia
epidermal
ultrasonography
podiatric
metastasis
contraceptive

ANSWER COLUMN

9-1

Dictionary
  practice

super- and supra- are both prefixes that mean above or beyond. Use your medical dictionary to analyze the following words in which super and supra- are used. Write the meaning of the word as you analyze its word parts.

9-2

	super-	**meaning**
super/fici/al	superficial	_____
super/cili/ary	superciliary	_____
super/infect/ion	superinfection	_____
super/ior/ity	superiority	_____

9-3

Refer to the illustration of the regions of the abdomen on p. 332.

	supra-	**meaning**
supra/lumb/ar	supralumbar	_____
supra/pub/ic	suprapubic	_____
supra/mammary	supramammary	_____
supra/ren/al	suprarenal	_____
supra/inguinal	suprainguinal	_____

More prefixes! Use this chart to work **Frames 9-4–9-27**.

Prefix	Meaning	Special Comment
epi-	over, upon	epicenter of an earthquake
extra-	outside of, beyond, in addition to	extracurricular activities
infra-	below, under	almost always below a part of the body
		almost always adjectival in form
		fewer words begin with infra- than with sub-
sub-	under, below	many words begin with sub-
meta-	beyond, after, occurring later in a series	also used with chemical names

ANSWER COLUMN

9-4

The epi/gastr/ic region is the region

over the stomach   *_____.

9-5

Epi/splen/itis means inflammation of the tissue

over the spleen   *_____.

Direction	Prefix	Word root/Suffix
below	hypo	chondr/iac
upon	epi	gastr/ic
above	supra	lumb/ar
below	hypo	gastr/ic

Thorax

1 Hypo-chondriac region	2 Epigastric region	1 Hypo-chondriac region
3 Lumbar region	4 Umbilical region	3 Lumbar region
5 Iliac region	6 Hypogastric region	5 Iliac region

Regions of the abdomen

9-6

Build a word meaning:
inflammation of the area over the bladder

epi/cyst/itis
ep′ i sis **tī′** tis

_____;

inflammation (of the tissue) on the kidney

epi/nephr/itis
ep′ i nef **rī′** tis

_____.

ANSWER COLUMN

9-7

Build a word meaning pertaining to
(the tissue) upon the skin (outermost layer)

epi/derm/al

_____ ;

(the tissue) covering the cranium

epi/crani/al

_____ ;

the area above the stern/um

epi/stern/al

_____ ;

the tissues on the heart

epi/card/ium
(You pronounce)

_____ .

9-8

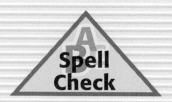

Information Frame

Recall that the **meninges** is a three-layered membrane surrounding the spinal cord and brain. The three layers include the pia mater, arachnoid, and the outermost layer the dura mater. Injuries to the head or spine may cause hematomas or hemorrhaging near these layers. A **sub/dural** hematoma is below the dura mater. An **epi/dural** hematoma is upon the dura mater.

9-9

An/esthesia may be administered near the dura mater of the spine (epidural) to block pain sensation to a specific area. This epi/dural an/esthetic may be used during childbirth, Cesarean section, or other surgery for pain control. If the anesthetic is injected upon the dura mater, it is _____ anesthetic.

epi/dur/al
e pi **der'** əl

9-10

Spell Check

Beware not to confuse "dural" with "dermal." Dura refers to the layers of the **meninges**. Dermal refers to the **skin**. Epi/dural is upon the dura mater. Epi/dermal is upon the dermis of the skin.

9-11

Extra- means outside of or beyond. Extra/nuclear means

outside of or beyond

* _____ the nucleus of a cell.

ANSWER COLUMN

9-12

outside of or beyond

Extra/uterine means *_____ the uterus.

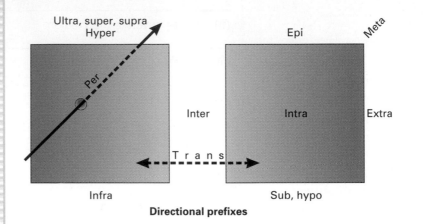

Directional prefixes

9-13

Build a word meaning outside of the:

joint

_____;

extra-/articul/ar
eks′ trə är **tik′** yə lər

urinary bladder

_____;

extra/cyst/ic
eks′ trə **sis′** tik

dura matter (meninges)

_____;

extra/dur/al
eks′ trə **door′** əl

genitals

_____;

extra/genit/al
eks′ trə **jen′** i təl

liver

_____;

extra/hepat/ic
eks′ trə hep **at′** ik

cerebrum

_____.

extra/cerebr/al
eks′ trə se **rē′** brəl

ANSWER COLUMN

	9-14
	Look at the words in the last frame. Draw a conclusion. extra- is used as a prefix in words that are usually
adjectives	_____ (nouns/adjectives).
	9-15
	infra- means below or under. Infra/patell/ar means
below or under	*_____ the patella (kneecap).
	9-16
	sub- is also a prefix that means
under or below	*_____.
	9-17
sub-	Below the tongue is _____ lingual.
	9-18
under	Sub/abdominal means _____ the
	abdomen. **aur** is one word root for ear. Sub/aur/al means
below	_____ the ear. Sub/cutaneous
below	(subcu, subq, s.c.) means _____
	the skin.
	9-19
	The prefixes infra- and sub- are sometimes confusing in word build-ing. For that reason, you will build words that can take either prefix. When you see sub- or infra-, you will think of
under	_____ or
below	_____.

9-20

Using **stern/o**, build two words meaning below the sternum.

infra/stern/al
in' fra **ster'** nəl
sub/stern/al
sub **ster'** nəl

_____ al

_____

A word meaning above the sternum is

supra/stern/al
sū' pra **ster'** nəl

supra _____.

9-21

Using cost/o, build two words meaning under the ribs:

infra/cost/al
sub/cost/al

_____ al,

_____.

A word meaning above the ribs is

supra/cost/al
(You pronounce)

_____.

9-22

Information Frame

meta- is a prefix used in many ways. Look at the table on page 331 to discover its meanings.

9-23

Analyze the term **metaphysics**. It is the study of things

beyond the physical,
   or the spirit

*_____

_____.

9-24

The bones of the hand that are beyond the carpals (wrists)

meta/carpals
met ə **kar'** palz

are the _____.

ANSWER COLUMN

meta/tarsals
met ə **tar'** salz

9-25

The bones of the foot that are beyond the tarsals (ankles)
are the _____.

meta/stasis
me **tas'** tə sis

9-26

A metastasis (metas., mets.) occurs when a disease spreads beyond
its point of origin. A metastatic (adjective) tumor is a secondary
growth from a malignant tumor. This secondary growth is a
_____.

metastasis

9-27

The area of the origin of cancer or the first discovered site in a
patient is said to be the "primary site."
If a "secondary site" is found, it may be a
_____.

ultra/violet
ul tra **vī'** ō let

9-28

ultra- is a prefix meaning beyond or in excess. Light waves that are
beyond the violet frequency are
_____ (UV).

ANSWER COLUMN

9-29

Sound waves that are beyond the audible frequency are ultra/son/ic. The process of making an image using ultrasound is called

ultra/son/o/graphy
ul′ tra son **og′** raf ē

_____.

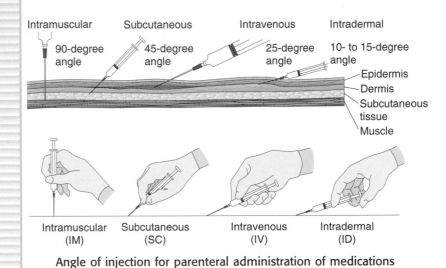

Intramuscular	Subcutaneous	Intravenous	Intradermal
90-degree angle	45-degree angle	25-degree angle	10- to 15-degree angle

Epidermis
Dermis
Subcutaneous tissue
Muscle

Intramuscular (IM)   Subcutaneous (SC)   Intravenous (IV)   Intradermal (ID)

Angle of injection for parenteral administration of medications

9-30

Ultrasound may be used for therapy or for diagnostic testing. To detect gallstones in a diseased gallbladder, the sonographer uses

ultrasonography

diagnostic _____.
To treat a patient with kidney stones, the sonographer

ultrasonography

uses therapeutic _____.

9-31

intra- means within. Intra-abdominal means

within the abdomen

* _____.

ANSWER COLUMN

9-32

within a cell   Intra/cellular means *_____.

within the uterus   Intra/uterine means *_____.

9-33

Using intra- and the adjectives ven/ous, spin/al, and lumb/ar, build a word meaning:

within a vein

intra/venous
in' tra **vē'** nus   _____ (IV);

within the spine

intra/spinal
in' tra **spī'** nəl   _____;

within the lumbar region

intra/lumbar
in' tra **lum'** bar   _____.

9-34

Build an adjective meaning:

within an artery

intra/arterial
in' tra är **tēr'** ē əl   _____;

within the cranium

intra/cranial
in' tra **krā'** nē əl   _____;

within the bladder

intra/cystic
in' tra **sis'** tik   _____.

9-35

Build an adjective meaning:
within the skin

intra/derm/al

_____ ;

within the duodenum

intra/duoden/al

_____ ;

within the thoracic cavity

intra/thorac/ic
(You pronounce)

_____ .

9-36

against

Contra/ry things are _____

each other. A contra/ry person is one who is

against

_____ your wishes.

9-37

In medical terminology, contra- is mainly confined in use to four
words. However, in these four words contra- still

against

means _____ .

9-38

Look up the words below in your dictionary:
contraindication

contra/indication
kon' tra in di **kā'** shun

_____ ;

contraceptive

contra/ceptive
kon' tra **sep'** tiv

_____ ;

contralateral

contra/later/al
kon' tra **lat'** ər əl

_____ .

ANSWER COLUMN

9-39

Using the words in **Frame 9-38**, fill the following blanks with a word whose literal meaning is:

against indication

contraindication

_____ (noun);

pertaining to against conception

contraceptive

_____ (adj.);

against the side

contralateral

_____ (adj.).

9-40

Recall that trans- is a prefix meaning across or over.
To trans/port a cargo is to carry it

across or over

* _____ the ocean or land.

9-41

Trans/position means literally position

across or over

* _____.

9-42

"Transposition" literally means placed across. When an organ is placed across to the other side of the body (from where it is normally found), _____ occurs.

trans/position
trans' pə **zi'** shun

9-43

Cardi/ac transposition means that the heart is on the right side of the body. If the stomach is on the right side of the body, the condition is gastr/ic _____.

transposition

9-44

When a trans/fusion is given, blood is passed

across or over

* _____ from one person to another.

ANSWER COLUMN

9-45

Analyze by drawing the diagonals.

trans/sexual

trans/illumin/ation

trans/vagin/al

trans/thorac/ic

trans/urethr/al

(You pronounce)

transsexual _____

transillumination _____

transvaginal _____

transthoracic _____

transurethral _____

9-46

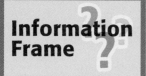

A catheter is a flexible tubular instrument. When a sterile urine specimen is needed, the urologist may introduce a catheter through the urethra into the bladder to obtain the specimen.
(Pronounced: **kath'** ə ter)

9-47

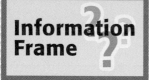

A procedure for enlarging heart vessels is called transcatheter therapy. It is possible to introduce an intravascular occlusion balloon "through" a catheter. Look up these terms in your dictionary and note the use of the prefix trans-.

9-48

retro- is a prefix meaning behind. Build an adjective meaning:
behind the colon

retro/col/ic

ret' rō **kol'** ik

_____ ic;

behind the mammary (gland; breast)

retro/mammary

ret' rō **mam'** ə rē

_____ mammary;

behind the stern/um

retro/stern/al

ret' rō **stûr'** nəl

_____ al.

ANSWER COLUMN

retro/version
ret' rō **vûr'** zhən

9-49

Version is turning or twisting. If ante/version means turning forward, then the word for turning backward is

_____.

9-50

behind

retro/periton/itis
ret' rō per i tə **nī'** tis

The **peritoneum** lines the abdominal cavity. The retro/periton/eum is the space _____ the peritoneum. An inflammation of this space is called

_____.

9-51

bending forward

flex/ion is bending or shortening of a body part (usually at a joint). ante- is the prefix for front or forward, therefore, the word ante/flexion means
* _____.

9-52

retro/flexion
ret rō **flek'** shən

ante/flexion

retro- means behind (or backward). Build a term meaning bending backward

_____;

bending forward

_____.

9-53

bending backward

bending forward

Retro/flexion of the uterus means the uterus is
* _____.

Ante/flexion of the uterus means
* _____.

ANSWER COLUMN

9.54

"Versio" is Latin for turning. The following words could have your head "turning" trying to keep them straight:

"version" word	Meaning
in/version	turning upside down
e/version	turning inside outward
a/version	turning away from, avoidance
ante/version	turning toward the front, forward
retro/version	turning toward the back, backward
con/vergence	turning toward each other (e.g., eyes)

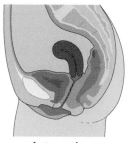 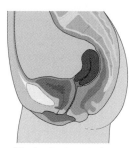 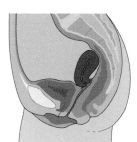

Anteversion   Marked retroversion   Retroflexion
Uterine Positions

9-55

If you have a sensation of turning or spinning when you are standing still, it is called **vertigo**. The word is built from **versio**, but the "s" changes to "t." Some people feel a dizziness that may be associated with an inner-ear disorder, and this spinning sensation is called
_____.

vertigo
ver' ti gō

9-56

os (oculus sinister) is the abbreviation for left eye. **sinistr/o** is the combining form for left. ad as a prefix or suffix means toward. Sinistr/ad means toward the _____.

left

ANSWER COLUMN

	9-57
	Using **sinistr/o**, build a word meaning:
	pertaining to the left
sinistr/al	
sin′ is trəl	_____ ;
	displacement of the heart to the left
sinistr/o/cardia	
sin′ is trō **kär** dē ə	_____ ;
	pertaining to the left half of the cerebrum
sinistr/o/cerebr/al	
sin′ is trō se **rē′** ə brəl	_____ .

	9-58
	Using manual (hand) and pedal (foot), build a word meaning:
	left-handed
sinistr/o/manual	_____ ;
	left-footed
sinistr/o/pedal	
(You pronounce)	_____ .

	9-59
	od (oculus dexter) is the abbreviation for right eye. The opposite of
right	**sinistr/o** is **dextr/o. Dextr/o** means _____ .

	9-60
right	Dextr/ad means toward the _____ .

	9-61
	Build a word meaning:
dextr/al	pertaining to the right _____ ;
dek′ strəl	displacement of the heart to the right
dextr/o/cardia	
dek′ strō **kär** dē ə	_____ ;
	displacement of the stomach to the right
dextr/o/gastria	
dek′ strō **gas′** trē ə	_____ .

ANSWER COLUMN

9-62

Refer to **Frame 9-61** if necessary and build a word meaning:

right-handed

dextr/o/manual

_____ ;

right-footed

dextr/o/pedal
(You pronounce)

_____ .

9-63

pod/o and **ped/i** are both combining forms for foot. Two terms for foot pain are

ped/i/algia
pe dē **al'** jē ə

_____ and

pod/algia
po **dal'** jē ə

_____ .

9-64

The two combining forms for foot are

ped/i
pod/o

_____ and

_____ .

9-65

Career Profile

Podiatrists (DPM) and podiatric assistants diagnose and treat diseases and disorders of the foot. This treatment may include surgery, prosthesis, and medical care for the foot. Assistants serve as office managers and clinical assistants performing medical office duties, x-rays, casting, and surgical assisting.

9-66

Suffixes -iatrist (noun) and -iatric (adjective) are used to indicate medical professionals. A health professional responsible for care of conditions of the feet is a

pod/iatrist
pō **dī'** ə trist

_____ (DPM).

ANSWER COLUMN

9-67

A hammertoe operation is a type of

pod/iatric
pō dē **ā′** trik

_____ (adjective)

treatment.

9-68

Look up **chirospasm;** it means

spasm of the hand
chir/o

*_____. The combining

form for hand is _____.

9-69

Chiropractors (DC) use their hands to manipulate the body for therapy. In the adjective chir/o/practic, the combining form

hands

chir/o means _____.

9-70

Surgical repair of the hand is called

chir/o/plasty
kī′ rō plas′ tē

_____.

9-71

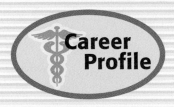
Career
Profile

Chiropractors (DC) and chiropractic assistants: Chiropractors are practitioners who use a system of treating disease by manipulation of the vertebral column and skull bones. This treatment is based on the theory that disease is caused by pressure on nerves and blood vessels because of faulty bone alignment. The assistants help the chiropractor with patients and perform administrative office procedures.

9-72

Spinal manipulation is a form of

chir/o/practic
kī′ rō **prak′** tik

_____ (adjective)

treatment.

ANSWER COLUMN

9-73

from or away from

ab- is a prefix that means *_____.

9-74

Ab/duct/ion means movement away from a midline.
When the arm is raised away from the side of the body,

ab/duct/ion
ab **duk'** shun

_____ has occurred.

9-75

Abduction can occur from any midline. When the fingers of the

abduction

hand are spread apart, _____
has occurred in four fingers.

9-76

ad- is a prefix meaning toward. Movement toward a
midline is _____.

ad/duct/ion
ə **duk′** shən

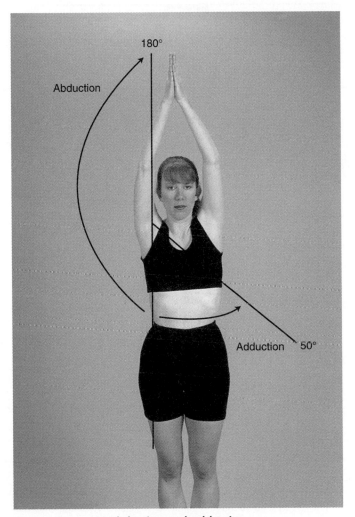

Abduction and adduction

9-77

"Addiction" means being drawn toward some habit.
The person who takes drugs habitually suffers from drug
_____.

ad/diction
ə **dik′** shən

ANSWER COLUMN

9-78

Addiction implies habit. Alcoholism is an

addiction

_____ to alcohol.

9-79

A person addicted to drugs is a drug addict. A person

addict

addicted to cocaine is a cocaine _____.

9-80

An ad/hesion is formed when two normally separate tissues join
together. They adhere to each other. Adhering to another

ad/hesion

ad **hē′** zhən

part forms an _____.

9-81

Patients are usually encouraged to ambulate soon after surgery to

adhesions

help prevent postoperative _____.

9-82

Pain or intestinal obstruction may be caused by

adhesions

abdominal _____.

Use the following information to work **Frames 9-83/9–102**. This is
another group of prefixes of place.

Prefix	Meaning	Differentiation
dia-	through	used with the word root for medical terminology
per-	through	prefix from Latin used more often in ordinary English
peri-	around	prefix from Greek used with the word root and combining forms for medical terminology
circum-	around	Latin prefix used more often in ordinary English

ANSWER COLUMN

9-83

Peri/articular means around articulations or joints.

around the tonsil

Peri/tonsill/ar means *_____.

9-84

around the colon or
   pertaining to
   around the colon

Peri/col/ic means *_____

_____.

9-85

Peri/odont/al means pertaining to diseases of the support structures around (peri) the teeth (odont/o). A word that means around a cartilage is

peri/chondr/al
per i **kon'** drəl

_____.

9-86

Build a word meaning:
inflammation around a gland

peri/aden/itis

_____;

inflammation around the vagina

peri/colp/itis

_____;

inflammation around the liver

peri/hepat/itis

_____;

excision of tissue (pericardium) around the heart

peri/cardi/ectomy
(You pronounce)

_____.

9-87

Cutting into the body is incision. Cutting out tissue is excision. Circum/cision (sur kum **si'** shun) cuts

around

_____ the foreskin of the penis.

ANSWER COLUMN

---

circum-
around

9-88

Another prefix that means around is
_____. Circum/ocular
means _____ the eyes.

---

around

9-89

Circum/or/al means _____ the mouth.

---

circum/scribed
ser' kəm skrīb'd

9-90

Circumscribed means limited in space (as though a line were drawn around it). A hive is limited in space—it has a defined area. A hive may be called a _____ wheal.

---

circumscribed

9-91

A boil is also limited in the space it covers. A boil is a
_____ lesion.

---

circumscribed

9-92

Pimples and pustules are also _____
lesions.

---

circum/duction
ser' kəm **duk'** shən

9-93

Moving toward is ad/duction. Moving away is ab/duction. Moving around (circular motion) is
_____.

ANSWER COLUMN

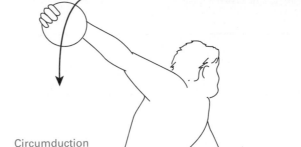

Circumduction

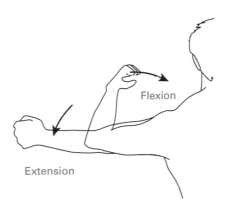

Flexion

Extension

9-94

Two prefixes mean through. The one that you would expect to use more often in medical terminology is _____.

dia-

9-95

You have already learned dia/gnosis, which means knowing _____, and dia/thermy, which means heating _____.

through
through

ANSWER COLUMN

9-96

dia/rrhea
dī ə **rē′** ə
dia/thermy
dī′ ə ther mē

Build a word meaning:
flowing through _____;

heating through _____.

9-97

Thinking frame
dia/phor/esis
dī ə fôr **ē′** sis

Diaphoresis is a condition of profuse sweating.
Diaphoretic is the adjectival form. Can you think of
the reason for using dia- as the prefix in these terms?

9-98

diaphoresis

Profuse sweating associated with acute myocardial
infarction (MI) is called _____

9-99

through

per- is a prefix meaning through. To per/for/ate (verb) means to
puncture or make a hole _____.

9-100

per/for/ated
per′ fōr ā t′d

The past tense of per/for/ate is per/for/ated. A
_____ (past tense) ulcer
is one that has eaten through the stomach.

9-101

per/for/ate
per′ fōr āt

Ulcers can also _____ (present
tense) the duodenum.

ANSWER COLUMN

9-102

Percussion (noun) means a striking through. Read the section on percussion in a dictionary. Analyze the word here.

per/cussion
per **kə′** shən

NOTE: A drum is a percussion instrument.

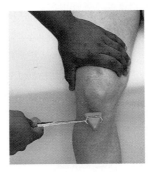

Assessment of Deep Tendon Reflexes

9-103

Information Frame

The following might be called the "Table of Con**fus**ion," but it will hopefully help you with medical terms ending in "-fusion". The combinig form **fus/o** is associated with melting or flowing together.

9-104

"Fusion" Term	Meaning
in/fusion	injecting fluids as into a vein
con/fusion	disturbed orientation as to time, place, person, or understanding
ef/fusion	escape of fluid into tissue, e.g., pleural effusion—fluid into the pleural space
per/fusion	pouring over or through, e.g., passage of blood through a vessel to the tissues

ANSWER COLUMN

9-105

A per/fusion/ist operates a heart–lung machine during open heart surgeries to ensure continued blood flow to the tissues even though the heart is not pumping. The patient will still have good tissue

per/fusion
per **fu′** zhən

_____.

9-106

The IV therapy team begins and monitors the administration of fluids intravenously. They may use an _____ pump, which controls the drip rate of the IV solutions.

in/fusion
In **fu′** zhən

9-107

Summarize: Two prefixes meaning through are _____ and _____. Two prefixes meaning around are _____ and _____.

per-
dia-
circum-
peri-

9-108

Look up the following terms in your dictionary. Notice that medical specialists use the word-building system to name new procedures. Write the meaning of each term.

through the skin
across the lumen
vessel repair

per/cutaneous *_____
trans/luminal *_____
angi/o/plasty *_____

9-109

para- means beside, beyond, near, abnormal, or indicates the lower half of the body.
"Paranephritis" means

inflammation near
  the kidney
inflammation near
  the liver

*_____.

"Parahepatitis" means *_____
_____.

ANSWER COLUMN

9-110

Using the prefix para-, build terms that mean:
inflammation near the bladder

para/cyst/itis
par ə sis tī tis
_____ ;

para/salping/itis
par' ə sal pin **jī'** tis

inflammation near the uterine tubes

_____ ;

near the vagina

para/vaginal
par' ə **va'** jin əl
_____ ;

near the uterus

para/uter/ine
par' ə **yōō'** ter in
_____ .

9-111

Paralysis is a loss of muscle function and sensation.

para/lysis
par **al'** ə sis
Para/plegia is _____ of the
lower body.

NOTE: Recall that peri- is also a prefix for around or near. Check your medical dictionary to see which terms are built using para- and which are built using peri-.

9-112

micro- means small. Hydro/cephalus is a condition involving fluid in the head. A condition of an abnormally small head is called

micro/cephalus
mī' krō **sef'** ə ləs
_____ .

9-113

Microcephalus limits the size of the brain. Most microcephalic people are mentally retarded. Occasionally, a baby is born with an unusually small head, or

microcephalus
_____ .

9-114

A cyst is a sac containing fluid. You also use **cyst/o** in building words pertaining to cysts.
A very small cyst is a

micro/cyst
mī' krō sist

_____.

A very small cell is a

micro/cyte
mī' krō sīt

_____.

The condition of having a small heart is

micro/cardia
mī' krō **kär'** dē ə

_____.

One-thousandth of a gram is a

micro/gram
mi' krō gram

_____.

9-115

Surgery performed on minute structures, using a microscope and small instruments, is _____.

micro/surgery
mī krō **sûr'** jər ē

9-116

macro- is the opposite of micro. Macro- is used in words to mean

large

_____.

9-117

Things that are macro/scop/ic can be seen with the naked eye.
Very large cells are called

macro/cyte(s)
mak' rō sīt(s)

_____.

ANSWER COLUMN

9-118

An abnormally large head is

_____.

macro/cephalus
ma′ krō **sef′** al us

A large cyst is a

_____.

macro/cyst
ma′ krō sist

A very large coccus is called a

_____ coccus.

macro/coccus
ma′ krō **ko′** kus

9-119

Define the following conditions.

abnormally:
  large tongue   macro/glossia   *_____
  large ear(s)   macrotia   *_____
  large nose   macro/rhinia   *_____
  large teeth   macro/dontia   *_____

9-120

homo- in words means same. Homo/genized milk has the same amount of cream throughout. Homo/glandular means pertaining to the *_____.

same gland

9-121

Homo/therm/al means having the _____ body temperature.

same (constant)

9-122

Homo/later/al means pertaining to the _____ side.

same

ANSWER COLUMN

9-123

Homo/sex/ual means being attracted to the same sex. When men are attracted to men more than to women,
they are said to be _____.

homo/sex/ual
hō′ mō **sek′** sho͞o əl

9-124

When women are attracted to women rather than to
men, they too are called _____.

homosexuals

9-125

hetero- is the opposite of homo-. hetero- means
_____.

different

9-126

Heter/ophthalm/ia means _____
color of each eye.

different

9-127

Heter/o/sex/ual means being attracted to a
_____ sex.

different

9-128

Look up the meaning of "homogeneous" and "heterogeneous." Draw the diagonal lines and write the definitions below:

_____

* _____ ;

_____

* _____ .

homo/gen/eous
hōm′ ō **jē′** nē us
pertaining to the
   same (tissues)
   throughout
hetero/gen/eous
het′ ûr o **jē′** nē us
pertaining to
   different (tissues)
   throughout

ANSWER COLUMN

9-129

Think of the meaning while you form **opposites** of the following:
homo/zyg/ous (twins from the same egg or zygote)

hetero/zyg/ous
het' er ō **zī'** gus

_____;

hetero/sex/ual
het' er ō **seks'** ū əl

homosexual

_____.

Prefix	Meaning	Explanation
semi-	half	Used with modern English words or words closer to modern English
hemi-	half	Used more often with straight medical words

9-130

semi-
hemi-

Two prefixes mean half. They are _____
and _____.

9-131

Form a word that means:

semi/circle
semi/conscious

half circle _____;
half conscious _____;
half private (hospital room)

semi/private

_____.

9-132

Build a word meaning:
presence of only half a heart (noun)

hemi/cardia
hem' i **kar'** dē ə

_____;

removal of half the stomach

hemi/gastr/ectomy
hem' i gast **rek'** tom ē

_____;

paralysis of half the body (on one side)

hemi/plegia
hem' i **plē'** jē ə or
hemi/paralysis
hem' i par **al'** ə sis

_____.

ANSWER COLUMN

9-133

Build a word meaning:

half circular

semi/circular

_____;

half normal

semi/normal

_____;

half comatose

semi/comatose
(You pronounce)

_____.

9-134

Information Frame ???

genit/o comes from the Greek word "genesis," meaning the beginning or formation. Structures of the reproductive system are called **genit/als.**

9-135

con- is a prefix that means **with** (c̄). Con/genit/al means

with

born _____.

9-136

A child with con/genit/al cataracts (opacity of the lens) was

born with

*_____ cataracts.

9-137

con/genit/al
kən **jen'** i təl

There are many con/genit/al deformities. A child born with a lateral curvature of the spine has _____ scoliosis.

9-138

Another way of saying a deformity that one is born with is to say **congenital anomaly**. A child born with kyphosis (posterior curvature of the spine) has a

congenital

_____ anomaly (abnormality).

ANSWER COLUMN

9-139

congenital

A child born with hydr/ophthalm/os has
_____ glaucoma (increased fluid
pressure condition of the eye).

9-140

congenital

A child born with syphilis has _____
syphilis.

9-141

dis- is a prefix that means to free from, to separate, or to undo.
Dis/ease literally means

free of ease

*_____.

9-142

To dis/sect is to cut a tissue or to undo it (into parts) for purposes
of study. Write the following forms of the word "dissect" below:
present tense verb

dissect or dis/sect/ing
dis **sekt'** ing

_____;

noun

dis/section
dis **sek'** shən

_____;

past tense verb

dis/sected
dis **sek'** td

_____.

9-143

In/ject means to introduce a substance into the body (usually
through a needle). Define the following:

verb form of inject
one who (thing
    which) injects
procedure of injecting
present tense verb
    inject
able to be injected

inject, injected *_____;
injector   *_____;

injection   *_____;
injecting   *_____;

injectable   *_____.

Information Frame

9-144

Fluids such as normal (isotonic) saline with 5% dextrose introduced into a vein is an IV infusion.

9-145

infusion

The pump used to regulate the speed of flow of an IV is called an _____ pump.

9-146

in/fus/ed
in/fus/ing
in/fus/able
in/fus/ion

From the word forms you learned with the word "inject," make the following forms of "infuse":
past tense   _____;
present tense   _____;
able to be infused _____;
noun   _____.

9-147

in/still/ation
in stil **ā'** shən

In Latin, "stillare" means to drop. A distiller condenses gases to form drops of liquid. Instillation is the process of administering drops of medication as into an eye or ear.
The physician ordered an _____ of antibiotic as treatment for the eye infection.

9-148

in/tolerance
in **tol'** er əns

Some people cannot tolerate various substances such as milk or sugar without having an unfavorable reaction. Two types of intolerance are lactose (from milk) and carbohydrate (from sugar) _____.

9-149

not

In **Frame 9-148**, the prefix in- means _____.

ANSWER COLUMN

9-150

Build a word meaning:

in/sane	not sane _____ sane;
in/somnia	inability to sleep _____ somnia;
in/continence	inability to control waste excretion _____ continence;
in/compatible	not compatible _____ compatible.

The following medical abbreviations correspond to the terms in Unit 9.

Abbreviation	Meaning
↑	above normal or elevated
↓	below normal or lowered
ac	antecibum (before meals)
c̄	with (cum)
CXR–PA & LAT	chest x-ray–postcroanterior and lateral views
DC	doctor of chiropractic
DPM	doctor of podiatric medicine
IM	intramuscular
IV	intravenous
LAT	lateral
mcg	microgram
metas., mets.	metastasis
MI	myocardial infarction
os	left eye
od	right eye
pc	post cibum (after meals)
po	postoperative
s̄	without (sum)
subcu., subq., s.c.	subcutaneous
UV	ultraviolet

You have been introduced to many new terms in this unit. To make sure you know them well, work the review exercises on the following pages. Also, listen to the CD-ROM accompanying the third edition of *Medical Terminology Made Easy* and practice pronunciation.

**UNIT 9
REVIEW EXERCISE**

Part 1: Review the terms you have learned in this unit by drawing the diagonal lines between the word parts and writing the meaning of each term. Use your medical dictionary or the frames if you need help. After you have completed these tasks, say each term aloud to practice pronunciation.

1. addiction _____
2. adduction _____
3. anteflexion _____
4. catheter _____
5. chiropractor _____
6. circumcision _____
7. circumscribed _____
8. contraceptive _____
9. contraindication _____
10. dextrocardia _____
11. diathermy _____
12. dissection _____
13. epidermal _____
14. epidural _____
15. epigastric _____
16. epinephritis _____
17. extranuclear _____
18. extrauterine _____
19. hemigastrectomy _____
20. hemiplegia _____
21. heteropia _____
22. homogeneous _____
23. hyperesthesia _____
24. infrapatellar _____
25. infrasternal _____
26. infusion _____
27. insomnia _____
28. intradermal _____

UNIT 9
REVIEW EXERCISES

29. intravenous _____

30. macrocytes _____

31. metacarpals _____

32. metastasis _____

33. microcephalus _____

34. parasalpingitis _____

35. percussion _____

36. perforated _____

37. perfusion _____

38. perichondral _____

39. peritonsillar _____

40. podalgia _____

41. podiatric _____

42. retroperitonitis _____

43. retroversion _____

44. semicomatose _____

45. semiconscious _____

46. subcutaneous _____

47. sublingual _____

48. superficial _____

49. supracranial _____

50. transurethral _____

51. ultrasonography _____

Part 2: Write the medical term that means:

1. tissues grown together _____

2. movement of a body part away from the body (noun) _____

3. making a circle with a body part _____

4. to make a hole through (verb) _____

5. to cut apart _____

6. instrument to view something small _____

7. person attracted to the same sex _____

UNIT 9
REVIEW EXERCISE

8. made up of different things_____

9. born with _____

10. put inside using a needle and syringe (noun) _____

Part 3: Match each term with its correct meaning.

_____ 1. sublingual
_____ 2. supralumbar
_____ 3. intramuscular
_____ 4. transposition
_____ 5. ultraviolet
_____ 6. inframammary
_____ 7. contraindicated
_____ 8. retroflexion
_____ 9. metatarsals
_____10. sinistromanual

a. to carry across to the other side
b. the bones beyond the wrist bones
c. light spectrum below red
d. light spectrum beyond violet
e. within the breast tissue
f. bending forward
g. bones beyond the ankle bones
h. below the tongue
i. placed across on the opposite side
j. between the skin
k. inside (or within) the muscle
l. above the lumbar spine
m. when a drug is advised against
n. left-handed
o. left-footed
p. below the breast
q. bending backward

Part 4: Prefix review. Draw a line from the meaning in the center to the correct prefix and suffix to complete the term. Then write the term in the answer blank. Write the term without using the hyphens.

Example:	sub	below the skin	cutaneous	subcutaneous
prefix		prefix word meaning	suffix	answer
contra-		1. placed across	-cyte	_____
hetero-		2. beyond violet light	-cardium	_____
homo-		3. not recommended for use	-flexion	_____
ad-		4. above the surface	-version	_____
peri-		5. same side	-position	_____
retro-		6. opposite sex attraction	-ficial	_____

**UNIT 9
REVIEW EXERCISE**

super-	7. around the heart	-sexual	_____
ultra-	8. large cell	-duction	_____
trans-	9. turned backward	-lateral	_____
macro-	10. movement toward	-violet	_____

Part 5: Define the following medical terms.

1. contraindication   _____

2. transposition   _____

3. intradermal   _____

4. ultrasonography   _____

5. metatarsals   _____

6. chiropractor   _____

7. podiatrist   _____

8. epidural   _____

Part 6: Match the abbreviations with their meanings.

_____1. c̄   a. intravenous

_____2. IM   b. lateral

_____3. LAT   c. intramuscular

_____4. DC   d. metastasis

_____5. DPM   e. before meals

_____6. IV   f. doctor of chiropractic

_____7. mets.   g. with

_____8. ac   h. doctor of podiatric medicine

Unit 9 Puzzle

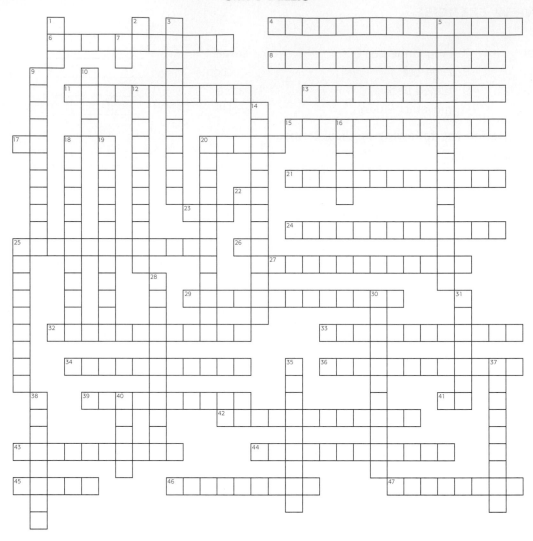

ACROSS

4. outside of a joint
6. pertaining to the tissues around the teeth
8. left-handed
11. origin (verb)
13. within the uterus
15. partially conscious
17. intravenous (abbrev.)
20. behind—suffix
21. above the groin
22. intramuscular
23. with—suffix
24. agent that prevents conception
25. within the skull
26. before meals
27. switched in position
29. abnormally small head
32. across (through) the vagina
33. heart displaced to the right
34. same side
36. inflammation near the bladder
39. one-sided paralysis
41. by mouth (per os)
42. through the skin
43. foot specialist
44. attracted to a different (opposite) sex
45. between—suffix
46. having a habit or compulsion to a substance
47. escape of fluid into tissues

DOWN

1. upon—suffix
2. toward—prefix
3. within the vein
5. recommended against (in certain circumstances)
7. left eye
9. turning forward
10. same as semi-
12. on the surface
14. move as to describe a circle
16. within—suffix
18. specialist who performs manipulation therapy
19. with the hands cut around e.g., removal of foreskin
19. cut around e.g., removal of foreskin
20. bending backward
25. turning upside down
28. hand bones beyond the carpals
30. beyond violet visible light
31. dizziness or spinning when still
35. joint movement away from the midline
37. introduced through a needle, e.g., medication
38. unable to sleep
40. large—prefix

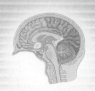

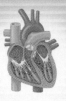

UNIT 10
Pathogenic Organisms, Endocrine System, and Medical Specialties

Study these word parts, meanings, and examples. Then proceed to the first frame.

COMBINING FORMS

adren/o (adrenal gland)
aer/o (air, with oxygen)
bacill/o (bacillus)
bi/o (life)
cocc/i (round-shaped bacteria)
cortic/o (cortex)
drom/o (running, a series)
endocrin/o (endocrine)
erg/o (work)
gen/o (forming, generating)
gluc/o (glucose)
glyc/o (glycogen, sweet)
gnos/o (to know, knowledge of)
immun/o (immune)
lys/o (destruction)
malari/o (malaria)
myc/o (fungus)
pharmac/o (drugs)
py/o (pus)
sept/o, seps/o (poisoned, toxic)
staphyl/o (growing in bunches)
strept/o (twisted chains)
test/o, orchid/o, orchi/o (testis)
thyr/o, thyroid/o (thyroid gland)

PREFIXES

a–, an– (without, lack of)
anti– (against)
dia– (through)
diplo– (two, double)
endo– (inside)
hyper– (above)
hypo– (below)
mal– (bad, poor)
poly– (too many)
pro– (before, in front of)
syn, sym– (joined, fused)

SUFFIXES

–crine (secrete)
–ism (theory, condition)
–ist (specialist)
–ity (ability)
–logy (study of)
–megaly (enlarged)
–pathy (disease)
–rrhea (flow, discharge)
–therapy (treatment)

Word Examples

COMBINING FORMS

adrenomegaly
aerobic
diplobacillus
biopsy
coccus
adrenocorticotropic
prodromal
endocrinologist
synergistic
pyogenic
glycolipid
diagnosis
immunodeficiency
glycolysis
malariotherapy
mycodermatitis
pharmacology
pyorrhea
septicemia
staphylococci
streptomycin
testicular
hypothyroidism

PREFIXES

asepsis
antiseptic
dialysis
diplococci
endocrine
hyperthyroidism
hypoglycemia
malnutrition
polyuria
prodrome
sympathectomy

SUFFIXES

exocrine
hyperthyroidism
pharmacist
immunity
endocrinology
immunology
thyroidomegaly
adrenopathy
pyorrhea
immunotherapy

ANSWER COLUMN

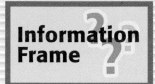

10-1

When a foreign invader (**antigen**) such as a bacteria or virus enters the body, specialized lymphocytes in the lymphatic tissues and blood-stream produce **antibodies** that disable the invaders. This antigen–antibody reaction is called the **immune response**. We even have a chemical memory so that the next time that same organism invades we have a quick defense. The body, either naturally or with the help of medical science, has several ways to develop an immune response. Study the following table.

Type of Immunity	Description
Natural immunity	Immunity we are born with as humans, e.g., dogs get canine distemper and humans do not.
Acquired immunity	Immunity the body develops in response to a foreign invader, such as bacteria or virus, or as a result of exposure through vaccination or antibodies.
Passive acquired immunity	Immunity passed from mother to infant or produced by injecting a person with antibodies from another source, e.g., gamma globulin, which helps boost the ability to fight off a possible infection.
Natural acquired immunity	Immunity in response to an acquired infection, e.g., chickenpox virus infection and illness usually occurs, antibodies are developed, and the person is protected against future exposures.
Artificially acquired immunity	Immunity in response to vaccination, e.g., MMR, measles, mumps, or rubella vaccine is injected and antibodies are developed, no illness occurs, and person is protected against future exposures.

10-2

immun/o/logy
im′ yōō **nol′** ō jē

immun/o is the combining form for immune. Immun/ity is one of the body's protections from diseases. The study of the function of the immune system is called _____.

ANSWER COLUMN

10-3

Immunization injections and oral preparations are given so a person may develop an immune response to certain diseases. The process is known as immun/o/therapy. DPT (diphtheria, pertussis, tetanus) and MMR (measles, mumps, rubella) are two types of

immun/o/therapy
im yōō′ nō **ther′** a pē

_____ or

immun/i/zations
im′ yōō nə **za′** shənz

_____ .

10-4

Immun/o/logists are studying the HIV (human immun/o/deficiency virus) virus that causes AIDS (acquired immunodeficiency syndrome). Because it is characterized by inability to fight off diseases, AIDS is a type of

immun/o/deficiency
im yōō′ nō de **fish′** en cē

_____ .

10-5

AIDS is called acquired immunodeficiency syndrome because an HIV infection is first acquired and then invades the immune system, interfering with the immune response. HIV infection is one cause of

immun/o/deficiency
im yōō′ nō dē **fish** en sē

_____ .

ANSWER COLUMN

10-6

Chickenpox is caused by a virus. When first infected, the person becomes ill. If infected again, the person will not likely become ill because of acquired active _____.

immun/i/ty
im **yoo'** ni tē

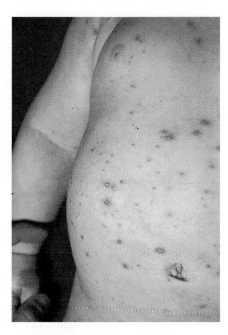

Varicella (Courtesy of Robert A. Silverman, M.D.,
clinical associate professor, Department of Pediatrics,
Georgetown University)

10-7

An infant being breast-fed receives antibodies from the mother's body through the milk. This process is called
passive _____.

immunity

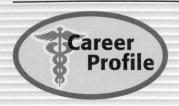

10-8

Biologists, biomedical engineers, geneticists, radiobiologists apply scientific principles and technology to provide understanding of physiologic and disease processes and to discover treatments.

RECOMMENDED CHILDHOOD IMMUNIZATION SCHEDULE
UNITED STATES, 2002

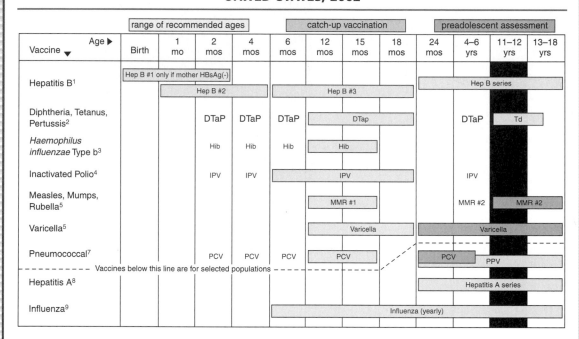

Vaccine ▼	Age ▶ Birth	1 mo	2 mos	4 mos	6 mos	12 mos	15 mos	18 mos	24 mos	4–6 yrs	11–12 yrs	13–18 yrs
			range of recommended ages				catch-up vaccination			preadolescent assessment		
Hepatitis B[1]	Hep B #1 only if mother HBsAg(-)		Hep B #2			Hep B #3				Hep B series		
Diphtheria, Tetanus, Pertussis[2]			DTaP	DTaP	DTaP	DTap				DTaP	Td	
Haemophilus influenzae Type b[3]			Hib	Hib	Hib	Hib						
Inactivated Polio[4]			IPV	IPV		IPV				IPV		
Measles, Mumps, Rubella[5]						MMR #1				MMR #2	MMR #2	
Varicella[5]						Varicella				Varicella		
Pneumococcal[7]			PCV	PCV	PCV	PCV			PCV	PPV		
Hepatitis A[8]										Hepatitis A series		
Influenza[9]					Influenza (yearly)							

Vaccines below this line are for selected populations

This schedule indicates the recommended ages for routine administration of currently licensed childhood vaccines, as of December 1, 2001, for children through age 18 years. Any dose not given at the recommended age should be given at any subsequent visit when indicated and feasible. ▮▮▮▮ Indicates age groups that warrant special effort to administer those vaccines not previously given. Additional vaccinces may be licensed and recommended during the year. Licensed combination vaccines may be used whenever any components of the combination are indicated and the vaccine's other components are not contraindicated. Providers should consult the manufacturers' package inserts for detailed recommendations.

Source: Approved by the Advisory Committee on Immunization Practices (www.cdc.gov/nip/acip), the American Academy of Pediatrics (www.aap.org), and the American Academy of Family Physicians (www.aafp.org).

ANSWER COLUMN

10-9

Explanation for
  next frame

In words such as "carcinoma" and "coccus," the first **"c"** is pronounced as a hard **"c"** or **"k"** sound. When followed by an **"o,"** **"u,"** or **"a"** or a consonant, a **"c"** is pronounced like a **"k"** sound.

10-10

hard **"c"** or **"k"**
  (pronounce them aloud)

In the words "colon" and "cardiac," the **"c"** is pronounced with a "*_____" sound.

10-11

Explanation for
  next frame

In the words "cerebrum" and "incision," the **"c"** is pronounced as a soft **"c"** or **"s"** sound. When **"c"** is followed by an **"i"** or **"e"** or **"y,"** it is pronounced with a soft **"c"** or **"s"** sound.

10-12

soft **"c"** or **"s"**

According to the **"c"** rule, in the words "cystocele" and encephalitis, each **"c"** is pronounced with a
*_____ sound.

10-13

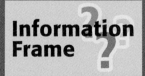

**Information
Frame**

Remember the **"c"** rule for those terms that follow with all of their **"c"'**s.

ANSWER COLUMN

	10-14
cocc	When building words about the spherically shaped family of bacteria, the cocc/i, use the word root _____.
	10-15
cocc/i **kok'** sī	Pneumonia may be caused by pneum/o/coccus. From this you know that the bacteria responsible for pneumonia belongs to the family _____ (plural).
	10-16
cocci	One form of meningitis is caused by the mening/o/coccus. It, too, is a member of the family _____ (plural).
	10-17
cocci **kok'** sī	There are three main types of cocci. Cocci growing in pairs are <u>diplo</u>_____.
	10-18
diplo/coccus dip' lō **kok'** us	Gon/o/rrhea is a venereal disease caused by *Neisseria gonorrhoeae*. This gon/o/coccus grows in pairs, so it is a _____.

ANSWER COLUMN

10-19

cocci

Cocci growing in twisted chains are
_____ strept o _____.

cocci

Cocci growing in clusters are
_____ strept o _____.

BACTERIA

Cocci

Bacilli

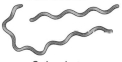

Diplococcus   *Staphylococcus*

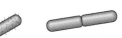

Bacillus   *Diplobacillus*

Curved rods

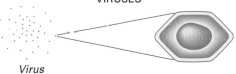

Spirochete   *Streptococcus*   *Streptobacillus*

VIRUSES

Virus

OTHER PATHOGENS

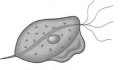
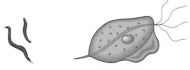
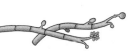

Filarial worms   *Trichomonas*   *Yeast*   *Lice*

Disease-producing Microorganisms

ANSWER COLUMN

10-20

strept/o means twisted chains or strips. Strept/o/cocci grow in twisted chains like this. If you see a chain of cocci when examining a slide under the microscope, you would say they were

strept/o/cocci
strəp' tō **kok'** sī

_____.

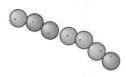

Streptococcus

10-21

Name the type of coccus in the following statements. Sore throat may be caused by beta hemolytic

strept/o/coccus
strəp' tō **kok'** us
Streptococcus

_____. Some pus formation
is due to _____ *pyogenes*.

10-22

"Staphyle" is the Greek word for bunch of grapes. **staphyl/o** is used to build words that suggest a bunch of grapes. Staphyl/o/cocci grow in clusters like a bunch of _____.

grapes

10-23

Staphylococci grow in clusters like grapes. If you see a cluster of cocci when using the microscope, you would say they were

staphyl/o/cocci
staf' i lō **kok'** sī

_____.

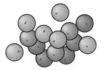

Staphylococcus

NOTE: Proper genus and species names are usually found italicized with the genus capitalized. When using the genus initial, it should also be capitalized. Examples: *Staphylococcus aureus*, or *S. aureus*.

ANSWER COLUMN

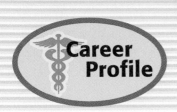

10-24

Medical technologists (ASCP-MT), medical laboratory technicians (MLT), and bioanalysts test blood, urine, other body fluids, and tissues to determine the presence of disease as well as administer diagnostic departments. They do research, teach and supervise technicians, and secure equipment and supplies.

10-25

The bacteria that cause carbuncles grow in a cluster like a bunch of grapes. Carbuncles are caused by

staphylococci

_____.

10-26

Most bacteria that form pus grow in a cluster.

staphylococci

They are _____.

10-27

Foods left unrefrigerated will grow bacteria that produces toxins. This common form of food poisoning is also caused

staphylococci

by _____.

10-28

Recall that **py/o** is the combining form used for words involving pus.

pus

A py/o/cele is a hernia containing _____.

10-29

Many staphylococci are pyogenic. A pus-producing bacillus is also

py/o/gen/ic
pī ō **jen'** ik

_____.

ANSWER COLUMN

10-30

A py/o/gen/ic bacterium is one that forms pus. You know the noun "genesis" for formation or beginning. The adjective that means something that produces or forms pus is _____.

py/o/gen/ic
pī ō **jen'** ik

10-31

Pyogenic bacteria are found in boils. Boils become purulent (contain pus). This pus is formed by _____ bacteria.

pyogenic

10-32

Py/orrhea means discharge of _____.

pus

10-33

Py/o/thorax means an accumulation of pus in the thoracic cavity. When pus-forming bacteria invade the thoracic lining, _____ results.

py/o/thorax
pī ō **thôr** aks

10-34

Pyothorax may follow chest disease. Pneumonia is one chest disease that can result in _____.

pyothorax

10-35

Look up **purulent** in your medical dictionary. It means pus forming or _____.

pyogenic

10-36

aer/o is used in words to mean air. You undoubtedly know the words aer/ial and aer/ialist. **Aer/o** always makes you think of _____.

air

ANSWER COLUMN

10-37

Using what you need of **aer/o**, build a word meaning:
abnormal fear of air

aer/o/phobia
air ō **fō'** bē ə

_____;

treatment with air

aer/o/therapy
air ō **ther'** ə pē

_____;

herniation containing air

aer/o/cele
air' ō sēl

_____.

10-38

bios is the Greek word for life. Bi/o/chemistry is the study of chemical changes in living things. The science (study of) living things is

bi/o/logy

_____.

10-39

A biologist is one who studies

living things or life

*_____ _____.

Biogenesis is the formation of

living things

*_____.

A biopsy (Bx) is a study of

living

_____ tissue.

Biochemistry is the study of chemical changes in

living

_____ things.

10-40

An an/aer/o/bic plant or animal cannot live in the presence of air
(an—without). Analyze anaerobic:

an-
aer/o
bic

prefix (without)   _____;
combining form (air) _____;
suffix (life)   _____.

ANSWER COLUMN

10-41

If anaerobic means existing without air (oxygen), build a word that means needing air (oxygen) to live (adjective):

aer/o/bic
air **ō′** bik

_____.

10-42

The bacterium that causes pneumonia requires air to live. These bacteria are considered _____ bacteria.

aerobic

10-43

Tetanus bacillus causes lockjaw. Lockjaw can develop only in closed wounds where air does not penetrate (e.g., stepping on an old nail). _Tetanus bacillus_ is an _____ bacterium. Read about tetanus in your medical dictionary.

an/aer/o/bic
an air **o′** bik

10-44

sepsis is a noun meaning a poisoned state caused by absorption of path/o/genic bacteria and their products into the bloodstream. A noun meaning a state without or free from sepsis is

a/sepsis
ā **sep′** sis

_____.

NOTE: Path/o/genic comes from **path/o** (disease), **gen** (forming), and **ic** (adjectival ending).

10-45

Sept/ic is the adjectival form of "sepsis." The adjectival form for the word meaning free from infection is

a/sept/ic
ā **sep′** tik

_____.

ANSWER COLUMN

10-46

Sept/i/cemia is an infection in the bloodstream.

infection with pus in
  the bloodstream

Sept/o/py/emia means *_____

_____.

NOTE: Toxic shock syndrome is caused by septicemia.

10-47

Study the last two frames. A combining form for infection

sept/o (used most)
  or seps/o
(You pronounce)

is _____.

10-48

Review the material from **Frames 10-44–10-46**.

seps/is
sept/ic
(You pronounce)

noun for infection   _____

adjective for infected   _____

a/seps/is

noun for state free from infection

_____

adjective for free from infection

a/sept/ic

_____

10-49

anti- is a prefix meaning against. An anti/pyretic is an agent that

against

works _____ a fever.

An anti/toxin is an agent that works

against

_____ a toxin.

NOTE: A toxin is a poisonous substance produced by an organism.

ANSWER COLUMN

10-50

The following is a table listing categories of drugs that work against something:

Drug Category	Works Against
anti/arrhythmic	irregular heartbeats
anti/arthritic	arthritis
anti/bacterial	bacteria
anti/biotic	bacteria
anti/cholinergic	parasympathetic impulses
anti/coagulant	blood clotting
anti/convulsive	seizures
anti/depressant	depression
anti/diarrheal	diarrhea
anti/emetic	vomiting
anti/fungal	fungi
anti/histamine	histamine (allergic reactions)
anti/hypertensive	high blood pressure
anti/-inflammatory	inflammation
anti/narcotic	narcotics
anti/neoplastic	tumors
anti/pruritic	dry skin (itching)
anti/septic	infective agents
anti/spasmodic	muscle spasms
anti/toxin	poisons (toxins)
anti/viral	viruses

10-51

An anti/narcotic is an agent that works ______________________ narcotics.

against

ANSWER COLUMN

10-52

An anti/biotic is an agent that works

against _____ bacterial infections.

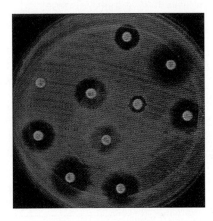

Antibiotic susceptibility test (C&S) plate showing clear areas
around antibiotic discs where bacterial growth is inhibited.

10-53

anti/biotic
(You pronounce)

Erythromycin is one type of _____.

10-54

Build a word describing the agent that works against:

anti/rheumatic
an ti rōō **ma′** tik
anti/spasmodic
an ti spaz **mod′** ik
anti/toxin
an ti **toks′** in

rheumatic disease _____;

spastic muscle _____;

toxins _____.

ANSWER COLUMN

anti/convulsive
an ti kon **vul'** siv
anti/arthritic
an ti ar **thri'** tik
anti/toxic
an ti **toks'** ik

anti/septic
an ti **sep'** tik

10-55

Build an adjective describing the agent that works against:
convulsive states _____ ;

arthritic diseases _____ ;

toxic states _____ ;

infection (against microorganisms)
_____ .

10-56

anti-/infectives
an ti in **fek'** tivz
anti-infectives

The major category of drugs that works against infection is
_____ . Disinfectants and
antiseptics, like iodine, are also
_____ .

10-57

Career Profile

Pharmacists (R.Ph) research, prepare, and dispense medications. They study the actions and interactions of medications and their effects on body function and in the treatment of disease. A pharmacist earns a minimum of a five-year baccalaureate degree and is licensed by each state. Pharmacy technicians assist pharmacists in preparing prescriptions, record keeping, and client services.

10-58

pharmac/o/logy
fär mə **ko'** lō gē

pharmac/ist
fär' mə sist

pharmac/o is the combining form pertaining to drugs. Use the word parts you have already learned to build a term that means:
the study of drugs
_____ ;

a drug specialist
_____ .

ANSWER COLUMN

10-59

Pneumon/o/myc/osis means a fungus disease of the lungs.
The word root that means "fungus" is _____.

myc

10-60

fungus (singular)
fung′ gəs
fungi (plural)
fun′ ji, **fun′** gī

myc/o, seen in a word, should make you think of
_____.

10-61

In high school biology, you read or learned the words **myc**elium and
mycelial. **Myc** refers to

fungi or fungus

* _____.

10-62

A mycosis is any condition caused by a fungus.
A condition of lung fungus is

pneumon/o/myc/osis
nōō′ mə nō mī **kō′** sis

_____.

10-63

Build a word meaning:
resembling fungi

myc/oid
mī′ koid

_____;

study of fungi

myc/o/logy
mī **kol′** ə jē

_____.

ANSWER COLUMN

pharyng/o/myc/osis
far in' gō mī **kō** sis

rhin/o/myc/osis
rīn' nō mī **kō** sis

dermat/o/myc/osis
derm ə tō mī **kō'** sis

myc/o/dermat/itis
mī' kō derm ə **tī'** tis

10-64

Build a word meaning:
fungus disease (condition) of the pharynx

_____;

fungus disease (condition) of the nose

_____;

fungus disease of the skin

_____;

inflammation of the skin caused by a fungus

_____.

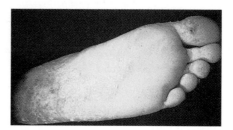

Tinea pedis (*Courtesy of the Centers for Disease Control and Prevention*)

SEXUALLY TRANSMITTED DISEASES (STDs)

Causative Agent	Disease
Bacteria	
Chlamydia trachomatis	Urogenital infection
Neisseria gonorrhoeae	Gonorrhea
Treponema pallidum	Syphilis
Viruses	
Hepatitis B virus (HBV)	Hepatitis
Human immunodeficiency virus (HIV)	AIDS (acquired immunodeficiency syndrome)
Human papillomavirus (HPV)	*Condylomata acuminata* (venereal warts)
Parasites	
Trichomonas vaginalis	Trichomoniasis
Phthirus pubis	Pediculosis pubis (crabs)
Sarcoptes scabiei	Scabies
Fungi	
Candida albicans	Candidiasis (yeast infection)

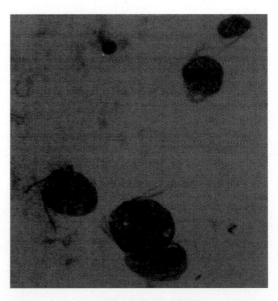

Trichomonas vaginalis

ANSWER COLUMN

10-65

Recall the prefix mal- means bad or poor. Look at the words in the next two frames. Now find the combining form for the disease

malari/o

malaria. _____

10-66

Before people knew that mosquitoes carry malaria and that it is caused by a parasite, they thought this disease was caused by "bad"

mal/aria (bad, air)
mə **lair'** ē ə

air. Analyze "malaria." _____

10-67

bad or poor

Mal/aise (mə lāz) means generally feeling *_____.

10-68

Although treatment exists, many people still have malaria. Analyze these words involving the disease malaria:

mal/ari/al
mal/ari/o/logy
mal/ari/o/therapy

malarial _____;
malariology _____;
malariotherapy _____.

10-69

syn- is a prefix meaning joined or fused. Syn/dactyl/ism means a joining of two or more digits. The prefix that means together,

syn-

joined, or fused is _____.

10-70

Syn/ergism occurs when two or more drugs or organs work together to produce an increased effect (syn-, join; **erg**, work; -ism, condition or state). Drugs that work together to increase each other's effects are called

syn/ergistic
sin er **jis'** tik

_____ (adjective) drugs.

ANSWER COLUMN

10-71

Syn/ergetic also means working (**erg**) together (**syn**), but usually it refers to muscles that work together. The three muscles in the forearm that work together are

syn/ergetic
sin er **je'** tik

_____ muscles.

10-72

APC tablets are frequently more effective for killing pain compared with aspirin alone. This is because aspirin, phenacetin, and caffeine

synergistic

are _____ drugs.

10-73

Analyze synarthrosis:

syn   prefix   _____;
arthr   word root (joint) _____;
osis   condition   _____.

10-74

Syn/arthr/osis indicates an immovable joint. The joining bones are fused together. When bones are fused at a joint so that there is no

syn/arthr/osis
sin är **thrō'** sis

movement, _____ occurs.
EXAMPLE: sacrum, pelvis

10-75

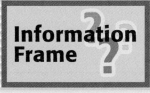

Information Frame

drom/o comes from the Greek word for "run." Drom/o/mania is an insane impulse to wander or roam. You usually use **drom** with the prefixes syn- and pro-.

ANSWER COLUMN

10-76

A syn/drome is a variety of symptoms occurring (running along) together. The complete picture of a disease is its

syndrome
sin' drōm

_____.

10-77

Look up "syndrome" in your dictionary. Read about Korsakoff's syndrome. Note some others. A syndrome due to alcoholism is

Korsakoff's syndrome
*_____

_____.

10-78

Expectant mothers are warned not to drink alcohol during pregnancy to prevent deformities in the newborn, known as fetal alcohol

syndrome
_____ (FAS).

10-79

Behavior changes and hyperemesis following a viral infection are symptoms occurring together that may indicate Reye's

syndrome
_____.

10-80

pro- is a prefix meaning before. Pro/drome means running before (a disease). Symptoms that indicate an approaching disease are its

pro/drome
prō' drōm

_____.

10-81

The sneezes that come before a common cold are the

prodrome
_____ of the cold.

ANSWER COLUMN

	10-82
prodromal	Chickenpox has a macular rash that precedes the papules. This is known as a _____ (adjective) rash.
	10-83
together or joined	syn- and sym- are different forms of the same prefix. syn- and sym- mean *_____.
	10-84
	You have already learned syn- in the words "syndactylism," "synergetic," "synarthrosis," and "syndrome."

	10-85
sym-	syn- is the form of the prefix used to mean fixed or joined, except when it is followed by the sound of **b, m, f, ph,** or **p.** Then _____ is used.
	10-86
suffering (medical) or feeling (standard)	"Sympathy" is an ordinary word that has a special medical meaning. Read this meaning in your medical dictionary. From either a medical or Webster's dictionary, find what it takes to fill this blank: sym- + **path/os**, the Greek word for _____.

ANSWER COLUMN

10-87

blephar/o means eyelid. A sym/physis is a growing together of parts. Sym/blepharon means *_____

eyelids have grown together, adhesions of the eyelids

_____.

10-88

pod/o is one combining form for "foot." Build a word meaning: lower extremities are grown together (united)

sym/podia
sim **pōd'** ē ə

_____ podia _____;

sym/path/ectomy
sim path **ek'** tom ē

excision of a sympathetic nerve
_____ path _____;

sym/path/oma
sim path **ō'** mə

tumor of a sympathetic nerve

_____.

10-89

Find a **common** word in your medical dictionary in which sym is followed by **m**. (There are only two or three to choose from.) One is

symmetry, symmetric,
or symmetrical

_____.

10-90

Find a **common** word in your medical dictionary that is used in ordinary English in which sym- is followed by **b**.

symbol or symbolism

*_____.

ANSWER COLUMN

b
m
p
f
ph

10-91

syn- and sym- both mean together. sym- is used when followed by the sound of the letters, _____, _____, _____, _____, and _____. syn- is used in other medical words.

Information Frame ??

10-92

In your dictionary, look up the word "gnosia." It comes from the Greek word meaning knowledge. Turn to the pronunciation key and read the **"g" rule**.

knowledge

10-93

The words **gnosia** and **gnosis** are medical words built from the Greek word meaning _____.

pro-

10-94

pro- is a prefix meaning in front of; **pro/gnosis** means foreknowledge, or predicting the outcome of a disease. The prefix that means "before or in front of" is _____.

pro/gno/sis
prog **nō′** sis

10-95

Leukemia is a serious disease associated with leukocytes. The _____ for acute leukemia is grave.

ANSWER COLUMN

10-96

"Procephalic" means in the front of the head. Analyze procephalic.

pro/cephal/ic
prō sə **fal'** ik
_____

"Prognostic" means giving an indication concerning the outcome of a disease. Analyze "prognostic."

pro/gnos/tic
prog **nos'** tik
_____

10-97

dia- means through. Dia/gnosis means

knowing through or
   know through
*_____.

10-98

dia/gnos/tic is the adjectival form of diagnosis, and dia/gnose is the

dia/gnos/tic
dī ag **nos'** tik
dia/gnose
dī' ag nōs
verb. When the results of the _____
(adjective) tests are complete, the physician will

_____ (verb) the condition of the
patient.

10-99

A diagnosis of a disease is made by studying **through** its symptoms.
When a patient tells of having chills, hot spells, and a runny nose, the

dia/gno/sis
dī əg **nō'** sis
physician may make a _____
of a head cold.

10-100

The literal meaning of dia/rrhea is

flowing through
*_____.

ANSWER COLUMN

10-101

Dia/thermy means generating heat through (tissues).

through   dia means   _____;

heat   **therm** means   _____;

suffix or ending   -y is a noun   * _____.

10-102

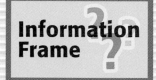

Dialysis is the separation of substances in a solution. Hemodialysis removes waste from the blood by using an artificial kidney.

10-103

Dialysis is a process of destroying waste products in the blood by diffusion **through** a membrane. People with kidney failure may

dia/lysis

dī **al'** i sis

need _____ to remove waste from their blood.

ANSWER COLUMN

10-104

Peritoneal dialysis and hemodialysis are two types of

dialysis

_____.

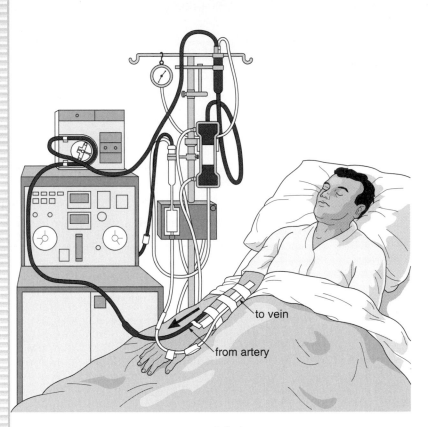

Hemodialysis

10-105

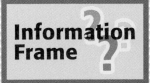

The endocrine system is made of several glands that secrete hormones. Its function is to work with the nervous system to regulate many body processes.

ANSWER COLUMN

10-106

The prefix endo- means inside. Endo/crine means to secrete inside. Hormones are secreted from the _____ glands.

endo/crine
en' dō krin

10-107

Hormone therapy is used to treat many diseases, such as diabetes mellitus. The medical specialty that is the study of the endocrine system is called _____.

endo/crin/ology
en' dō krin **o'** lō jē

10-108

The table below analyzes word parts related to the endocrine system. Refer to the illustration on the next page.

Combining Form	Meaning	Example
thyroid/o, thyr/o	thyroid gland	thyroidectomy
thym/o	thymus gland	thymosin
adren/o	adrenal gland	adrenalin
pancreat/o	pancreas	pancreatitis
oophor/o	ovary	oophoroma
test/ic/o, orchid/o, orchi/o	testis	testicular

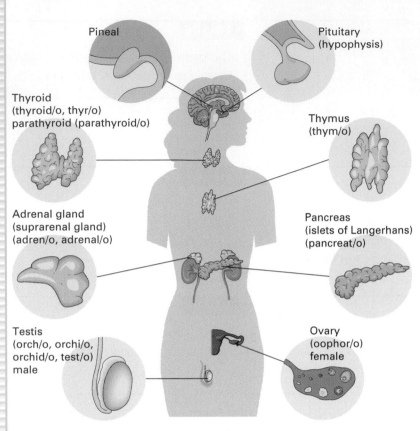

Pineal

Pituitary
(hypophysis)

Thyroid
(thyroid/o, thyr/o)
parathyroid (parathyroid/o)

Thymus
(thym/o)

Adrenal gland
(suprarenal gland)
(adren/o, adrenal/o)

Pancreas
(islets of Langerhans)
(pancreat/o)

Testis
(orch/o, orchi/o,
orchid/o, test/o)
male

Ovary
(oophor/o)
female

Structures of the Endocrine System

10-109

Analyze the following hormones and name the gland by which they
are produced:

adren/o/corticoid (cortisone)

adrenal gland
  (adrenal cortex)

* _____ ;

thyr/o/xin

thyroid gland

* _____ ;

test/o/sterone

testes

_____ .

See how much you have learned about word building!

ANSWER COLUMN

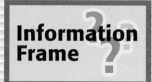

Information Frame

10-110

Locate the pancreas on the diagram of the endocrine system. The pancreas is a glandular organ in which the islets of Langerhans are located. Normally these glands secrete the hormone insulin, which affects the cell membrane, allowing the transportation of glucose (sugar) from the blood into the cells where it can be used. Most cells require the presence of insulin to be able to receive glucose. If a person does not produce enough or any insulin, the glucose level in the blood rises to abnormal levels. If there is too much insulin secreted, the blood glucose levels fall below normal.

10-111

An abnormally low blood-glucose level is called hypo/glyc/emia. **glyc/o** refers to sugar.

low

glucose

Hypo/glyc/emia means a _____ level of _____ in the blood.

10-112

Recall that hyper- means above normal. Build a word that means a high level of glucose in the blood:

hyper/glyc/emia

hī per glī **sē′** mē ə

_____.

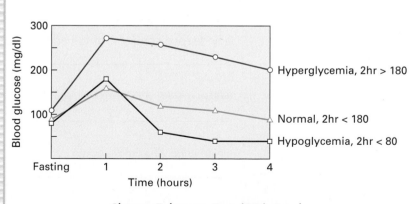

Glucose Tolerance Test (GTT) Graph

ANSWER COLUMN

10-113

Diabetes mellitus is a disease in which the body does not produce enough insulin. With a low level of insulin, the person will experience

hyperglycemia

the effects of _____.

10-114

poly- means too many or too much. Three symptoms common to people experiencing hyperglycemia are polyphagia, polydipsia, and polyuria. They are called the three "p's" of diabetes. From what you recall about these terms, indicate the meaning of each below. If not, look them up in your dictionary.

frequent urination   poly/uria   _____

abnormal increase in thirst   poly/dips/ia   _____

abnormal increase in hunger   poly/phagia   _____

10-115

Hyper/thyroid/ism is an overactive thyroid. An underactive (slow-acting) thyroid condition is called

hypo/thyroid/ism

hī pō **thī'** roid izm

_____.

10-116

Build a term meaning:
any disease condition of the adrenal glands

adren/o/pathy

ad rēn **o'** path ē

_____;

enlargement of the adrenal glands

adren/o/megaly

ad rēn ō **meg'** əl ē

_____;

destruction of adrenal tissue

adren/o/lysis

ad rēn **o'** li sis

_____.

ANSWER COLUMN

10-117

The adrenal glands also are called the supra/renal glands because they are above the kidneys. Epi/nephr/ine is a hormone produced by the supra/renal glands. Define these two terms:

above the kidneys
a hormone produced
  by glands located upon
  the kidney

supra/renal * _____ ;
epi/nephr/ine * _____
_____ .

10-118

glyc/o comes from the Greek word for "sweet." Glycogen is "animal starch" formed from simple sugars. The cells of the body use a simple sugar, glucose, to release energy. To use its reserve fuel supply of animal starch, the body must convert

glyc/o/gen
glī' kō jen

_____ to glucose.

10-119

Glucose is used by the muscles to release energy. Glycogen is the reserve food supply of glucose. Glucose is the usable form from the

glycogen

reserve supply of _____ .

10-120

Glycogen is potential sugar. Glucose is usable sugar. In words, **glyc/o**

sugar or sweet

should make you think of * _____ .

10-121

Glyc/emia means sugar in the blood. A symptom of diabetes is hyper/glyc/emia. This means * _____

too much sugar in
  the blood (high
  blood sugar)

_____ .

ANSWER COLUMN

10-122

Hyper/glyc/emia means high blood sugar. The word that means low blood sugar is _____.

hypo/glyc/emia
hī′ pō glī **sē′** mē ə

10-123

When a person produces too much insulin, the blood glucose level may decrease to below normal. This is called _____.

hypoglycemia

10-124

Recall that -lysis is the suffix for destruction. The breakdown (destruction) of glycogen is _____.
-rrhea is a suffix meaning flow or discharge. The discharge (flow) of sugar from the body is _____.

glyc/o/lysis
glī **kol′** ə sis
glyc/o/rrhea
glī kō **rē′** ə

10-125

Many hormones are produced by the pituitary gland. Look up pituitary in your dictionary and read about its function. The pituitary gland (hypophysis) has front and back lobes. These are called the _____ lobe (front) and the _____ lobe (back).

anterior
posterior

You have reached the end of your word-building system study of medical terminology. Each of these medical specialties uses medical terminology. Using your knowledge of word-building systems, complete the following chart. Using the numbers in each column, check your answers on the chart that follows.

Specialty	Specialist	Limits of Field
pathology	10-126	diseases—nature and causes
10-127	dermatologist	10-128
neurology	10-129	nervous system diseases
10-130	gynecologist	female diseases
urology	10-131	male diseases and all urinary diseases
10-132	endocrinologist	glands of internal secretion
oncology	10-133	neoplasms (new growths)
10-134	10-135	heart
ophthalmology	10-136	eye
10-137	otorhinolaryngologist	10-138
obstetrics	10-139	pregnancy, childbirth, and puerperium
10-140	geriatrician	old age
pediatrics	10-141	children
orthopedics	orthopedist	bones and muscles
psychiatry	10-142	mental disorders
10-143	audiologist	hearing function
radiology	10-144	diagnostic imaging, therapeutic x-ray
10-145	chiropractor	10-146
10-147	podiatrist	diseases of the foot

Answers

dermatology (10-127)

gynecology (10-130)

endocrinology (10-132)

cardiology (10-134)

pathologist (10-126)

neurologist (10-129)

urologist (10-131)

oncologist (10-133)
cardiologist (10-135)

skin (10-128)

Answers

Specialty	Specialist	Limits of Field
	ophthalmologist (10-136)	
otorhinolaryngology (10-137)		ear-nose-throat (10-138)
	obstetrician (10-139)	
geriatrics (10-140)		
	pediatrician (10-141)	
	psychiatrist (10-142)	
audiology (10-143)		
	radiologist (10-144)	
chiropractic (10-145)		manipulation therapy (10-146)
podiatry (10-147)		

See, you are now competent in systematic medical terminology, so

_____.

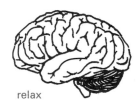

relax

You can proudly say that you have now completed this introductory study of medical terminology.

The following medical abbreviations correspond to the terms in Unit 10.

Abbreviation	Meaning
ACTH	adrenocorticotropic hormone
AIDS	acquired immunodeficiency syndrome
APC	aspirin, phenacetin, caffeine
Bx	biopsy
DC	doctor of chiropractic

ANSWER COLUMN

Abbreviation	Meaning
DPM	doctor of podiatric medicine
DTaP, DTP	diphtheria, pertussis, tetanus
Dx	diagnosis
FAS	fetal alcohol syndrome
FSH	follicle stimulating hormone
Hep B	hepatitis B vaccine
Hib	*Haemophilus influenzae* bacteria
HIV	human immunodeficiency virus
HPV	human papillomavirus
Hx	history
IDDM, Type I	insulin-dependent diabetes mellitus
IgG, IgM, IgE	immunoglobulins
IPV	inactivated polio vaccine
LH	leutinizing hormone
MMR	measles, mumps, rubella (vaccine)
MSH	melanocyte stimulating hormone
NIDDM	non-insulin-dependent diabetes mellitus
Px	prognosis
RPh	registered pharmacist
Rx	prescribe (take)
SIDS	sudden infant death syndrome
Staph	staphylococcus
STH	somatotropic hormone
STI	sexually transmitted infections
Strep	streptococcus
Sx	symptoms
T_3, T_4	thyroid hormones
Td	tetanus vaccine
TSH	thyroid stimulating hormone
Tx	treatment
Var	*Varicella* (chickenpox)

To complete your study, work the review exercises on the following pages. Also, listen to the CD-ROM accompanying the third edition of *Medical Terminology Made Easy* and practice pronunciation.

UNIT 10
REVIEW EXERCISE

Part 1: Review the terms you have learned in this unit by drawing the diagonal lines between the word parts and writing the meaning of each term. Use your medical dictionary or the frames if you need help. After you have completed these tasks, say each term aloud to practice pronunciation.

1. adrenocorticoid _____
2. adrenomegaly _____
3. aerobic _____
4. aerocele _____
5. aerophobia _____
6. anaerobic _____
7. antibiotic _____
8. anti-infective _____
9. antinarcotic _____
10. antiseptic _____
11. asepsis _____
12. biologist _____
13. chiropractic _____
14. dermatomycosis _____
15. diagnostic _____
16. dialysis _____
17. diplococci _____
18. disinfectant _____
19. endocrinologist _____
20. endocrinology _____
21. hyperglycemia _____
22. hyperthyroidism _____
23. hypoglycemia _____
24. immunization _____
25. immunodeficiency _____
26. immunology _____
27. immunotherapy _____

**UNIT 10
REVIEW EXERCISE**

28. malabsorption _____

29. malaise _____

30. malariotherapy _____

31. malnutrition _____

32. mycodermatitis _____

33. orthopedist _____

34. otorhinolaryngologist _____

35. pathologist _____

36. pediatrician _____

37. pneumococcus _____

38. pneumomycosis _____

39. podiatry _____

40. polydipsia _____

41. polyuria _____

42. prodromal _____

43. prognosis _____

44. pyogenic _____

45. pyorrhea _____

46. radiologist _____

47. septicemia _____

48. staphylococci _____

49. streptococcus _____

50. symmetry _____

51. sympodia _____

52. synarthrosis _____

53. syndrome _____

54. synergistic _____

55. testosterone _____

56. thyroidectomy _____

**UNIT 10
REVIEW EXERCISE**

Part 2: Match each term with its correct meaning.

_____ 1. immunologist

_____ 2. streptococcus

_____ 3. anaerobic

_____ 4. septopyemia

_____ 5. diplococcus

_____ 6. antibiotic

_____ 7. aerophobia

_____ 8. HIV

_____ 9. dermatomycosis

_____ 10. antiseptic

a. agent that works against toxins and pathogens

b. agent that works to promote the growth of bacteria in cultures

c. agent that prevents pregnancy

d. agent that prevents the growth of bacteria

e. fear of being alone

f. acute immunodisease syndrome

g. round-shaped bacteria growing in twisted chains

h. rod-shaped bacteria growing in bunches

i. pus producing infection in the blood

j. flow or discharge of pus

k. organism capable of growing without oxygen

l. fungus infection of the skin

m. fear of air

n. specialist in diseases of the endocrine system

o. specialist in resistance to disease

p. human immunodeficiency virus

q. round-shaped bacteria growing in pairs

Part 3: Write the medical term that means:

1. effect of greater strength than the sum of two drugs _____

2. joined feet _____

3. enlargement of the adrenal glands _____

4. predicting the outcome of a disease _____

5. symptoms that come before the onset of a disease _____

6. parasitic disease of the blood carried by mosquitoes _____

7. overactive thyroid condition _____

8. male hormone produced by the testes _____

9. physician specialist in hormone therapy _____

10. ear, nose, and throat specialist _____

UNIT 10
REVIEW EXERCISE

Part 4: Use the medical terms listed below to complete these sentences:

malnutrition	endocrinologist	immunodeficiency	aerobic	
antibiotic	fungus	streptococcus	staphylococcus	
pyorrhea	biopsy	insulin	dietitian	aseptic
septicemia	immunity	pyogenic	malaria	syndrome
prognosis	diagnosis	dialysis	adrenopathy	endocrine
oncologist	pathologist	dermatologist	neurologist	

1. After Chelsea was diagnosed with diabetes, she was counseled by a _____ about her food intake and exercise plan and was treated with _____ ordered by the _____.

2. A suspicious skin growth was noticed upon examination by the _____. He ordered an excision with _____ to determine whether or not it was cancerous.

3. Toxic shock _____ is really an infection that spreads to the blood-stream. It is called _____.

4. Dr. P. Brainard, the _____, ordered an EEG on his patient with a _____ of cephalalgia. Medication and biofeedback stress reduction tech-niques were prescribed for a favorable _____.

5. The HIV-positive child's ability to build _____ to disease was compromised as the acquired _____ progressed.

Part 5: Draw a line to match the abbreviation with its meaning.

1.	Bx	measles, mumps, rubella vaccine
2.	Rx	inactivated polio vaccine
3.	Tx	thyroid-stimulating hormone
4.	Dx	biopsy
5.	SIDS	human papillomavirus
6.	IPV	prescribe
7.	Hx	sudden infant death syndrome
8.	TSH	history
9.	MMRV	diagnosis
10.	HPV	treatment

UNIT 10
REVIEW EXERCISE

Part 6: Label the structures of the endocrine system using the following terms:

pineal gland	testis	thyroid gland
adrenal gland	ovary	pancrea
pituitary gland	thymus gland	

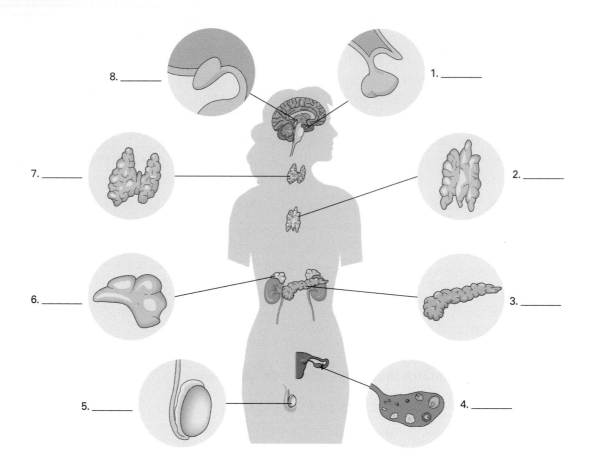

8. _____

1. _____

7. _____

2. _____

6. _____

3. _____

5. _____

4. _____

Unit 10 Puzzle

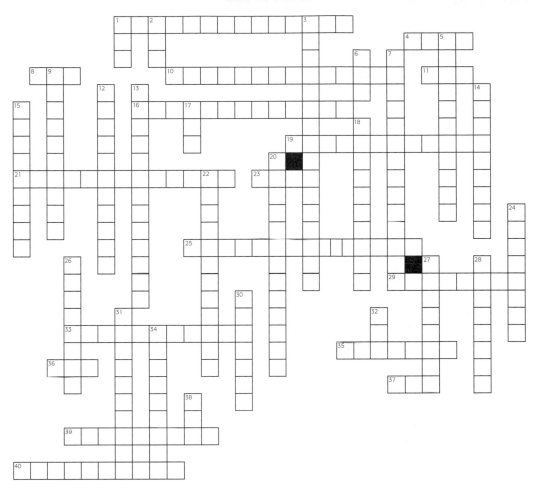

ACROSS

1. slow-acting thyroid
4. insulin-dependent diabetes mellitus
8. inactivated polio vaccine (abbrev.)
10. agent that works against seizures
11. doctor of podiatric medicine
16. excision of the thyroid gland
19. male sex hormone
21. high blood sugar
23. prefix for against
25. specialist in the endocrine system
29. symptoms occurring together
33. hormone produced by the adrenal medulla
35. blood parasite carried by mosquitoes
36. human immunodeficiency virus
37. varicella (chickenpox) vaccine
39. adrenal cortex hormone
40. specialist in drug therapy

DOWN

1. hepatitis B vaccine (abbrev.)
2. prefix for pus
3. lack of immunity
5. round bacterium in pairs
6. prefix for life
7. fungal infection of the skin
9. frequent thirst
12. working together
13. cocci growing in bunches
14. living without air
15. heating through tissues
17. registered pharmacist
18. frequent hunger
20. study of hormones
22. vaccination
24. even on both sides (nouns)
26. producting pus
27. front
28. frequent urination
30. free of poisons or toxins
31. agent that fights infection
32. prefix for bad
34. predicting the outcome of a disease
38. prefix for joined

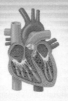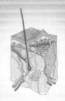

APPENDIX A
Weights and Measures, Chemical Symbols, Charting Abbreviations

Cover the abbreviation. Then read the meaning and write the abbreviation in the blank. Check your answer for accuracy.

WEIGHTS AND MEASURES

METRIC

kg	kilogram(s) (1000 g)	_____
hg	hectogram (100 g)	_____
dag	decagram (10 g)	_____
gm or g	gram	_____
dg	decigram (0.1 g)	_____
cg	centigram (0.01 g)	_____
mg	milligram (0.001 g)	_____
mcg	microgram (0.001 mg)	_____

STANDARD

lb, #	pound	_____
oz, 3	ounce	_____
dr, 3	dram	_____
gr	grain	_____

VOLUME

cu mm	cubic millimeter (mm^3)	_____
cc	cubic centimeter (cm^3)	_____
cu m	cubic meter (m^3)	_____
cu in	cubic inch (in^3)	_____
cu ft	cubic foot (ft^3)	_____
cu yd	cubic yard (yd^3)	_____

APOTHECARY

ī, īī, īīī   one, two, three   _____

īV, V̄, etc.   four, five, etc.   _____

īss   one and one-half   _____

LENGTHS

in, "   inch (2.54 cm)   _____

ft, '   foot (12 in)   _____

yd   yard (36 in)   _____

mm   millimeter (0.001 m)   _____

cm   centimeter (0.01 m)   _____

m   meter   _____

km   kilometer (1000 m)   _____

LIQUID VOLUME

t, tsp   teaspoon   _____

T, Tbsp   tablespoon   _____

c   cup   _____

m, min   minim   _____

ml   milliliter (0.001 L)   _____

cc   cubic centimeter (1 ml)   _____

cl   centiliter (0.01 L)   _____

dl   deciliter (0.1 L)   _____

L   liter (1000 ml)   _____

dal   decaliter (10 L)   _____

hl   hectoliter (100 L)   _____

fl dr, fl 3   fluid dram (60 min)   _____

fl oz, fl 3   fluid ounce (8 fl dr)   _____

pt   pint (16 oz)   _____

qt   quart (32 oz)   _____

gal,°   gallon (4 qt)   _____

gt   drop (1 min)   _____

gtt   drops   _____

MISCELLANEOUS

at wt   atomic weight   _____

C, kcal   calorie   _____

c, Ci   curie   _____

ht   height   _____

mA	milliampere	_____
mEq	milliequivalent	_____
MHz	megahertz	_____
mg%	milligram percent	_____
mw	molecular weight	_____
IU	international units	_____
U	units	_____
°C	degrees Celsius	_____
°F	degrees Fahrenheit	_____

CHEMICAL SYMBOLS

Al	aluminum	_____
Ar	argon	_____
As	arsenic	_____
Ba	barium	_____
B	boron	_____
Br	bromine	_____
Ca	calcium (Ca^{2+} ion)	_____
Cd	cadmium	_____
C	carbon	_____
CO_2	carbon dioxide	_____
pCO_2	partial pressure carbon dioxide	_____
Cl	chlorine (Cl^- ion)	_____
Cr	chromium	_____
Co	cobalt	_____
Cu	copper (Cu^{++} ion)	_____
F	fluorine	_____
$C_6H_{12}O_6$	glucose	_____
He	helium	_____
H	hydrogen	_____
H_2O	water	_____
I	iodine (I^{131} radioactive)	_____
Fe	iron (ferrum–Latin)	_____
K	potassium (kalium–Latin)	_____
Kr	krypton	_____
Pb	lead (plumbum–Latin)	_____
Li	lithium	_____

Mg	magnesium	_____
Mn	manganese	_____
Hg	mercury (hydragyrum—Latin)	_____
Ne	neon	_____
N	nitrogen	_____
O	oxygen (O_2)	_____
P	phosphorus	_____
pO_2	partial pressure oxygen	_____
Ra	radium	_____
Se	selenium	_____
Si	silicon	_____
Ag	silver (argentum—Latin)	_____
$AgNO_3$	silver nitrate	_____
Au	gold	_____
Na	sodium (natrium—Latin)	_____
NaCl	sodium chloride	_____
S	sulfur	_____
U	uranium	_____
Zn	zinc	_____

CHARTING ABBREVIATIONS

aa	of each	_____
AA	aortic aneurysm	_____
ac	before meals (antecibum)	_____
AD	right ear (auris dextra)	_____
ADL	activities of daily living	_____
adm	admission	_____
AJ	ankle jerk	_____
am	before noon (ante meridiem)	_____
AMA	against medical advice	_____
AMB	ambulate	_____
ant	anterior	_____
AP	anteroposterior	_____
approx	approximately	_____
AS or LE	left ear (auris sinistra)	_____
AV	atrioventricular	_____

bid	twice a day (bis in die)	_____
bin	twice a night (bis in nocte)	_____
BM	bowel movement	_____
BMR	basal metabolic rate	_____
BP	blood pressure	_____
BRP	bathroom privileges	_____
c̄	with (cum—Latin)	_____
C1, C2, C3 . . . C7	cervical vertebrae first, second, third . . . seventh	_____
C	centigrade, celsius, or large calorie (kilocalorie)	_____
cap(s)	capsule(s)	_____
CBR	complete bed rest	_____
CC	chief complaint	_____
CCU	cardiac care unit (coronary care unit)	_____
c/o	complains of	_____
cont	continue	_____
D	diopter (ocular measurement)	_____
dc	discontinue	_____
DC	discharge from hospital	_____
DNA	deoxyribonucleic acid	_____
DNR	do not resuscitate	_____
DNS	did not show	_____
Dr	doctor	_____
DTaP	diphtheria, tetanus, pertussis	_____
Dx	diagnosis	_____
EOM	extraocular movement	_____
ER	emergency room	_____
Ex	examination	_____
F	Fahrenheit	_____
FHS	fetal heart sounds	_____
FHT	fetal heart tones	_____
GB	gallbladder	_____

GI	gastrointestinal	_____
GU	genitourinary	_____
h, hr, °	hour	_____
Hct	hematocrit	_____
HEENT	head, ear, eye, nose, throat	_____
Hep B	hepatitis B vaccine	_____
Hgb, Hb	hemoglobin	_____
hpf	high power field	_____
HPV	human papillomavirus	_____
hs	hour of sleep, bedtime (hora somni)	_____
hypo	hypodermic injection	_____
ICU	intensive care unit	_____
IDDM, Type I	insulin-dependent diabetes mellitus	_____
IM	intramuscular	_____
I+O	intake and output	_____
IPV	inactivated polio vaccine	_____
$\overline{\text{iss}}$	one and one half	_____
IUD	intrauterine device	_____
IV	intravenous	_____
L	left	_____
L1, L2, L3 . . . L5	lumbar vertebrae first, second, third . . . fifth	_____
L+A	light and accommodation	_____
L+W	living and well	_____
LLQ	left lower quadrant	_____
LMP	last menstrual period	_____
LOA	left occipitoanterior	_____
LPF	low power field (10×)	_____
LUQ	left upper quadrant of abdomen	_____
MRI	magentic reasonance imaging	_____
MTD	right eardrum (membrana tympani dexter)	_____

MTS	left eardrum (membrana tympani sinister)	_____
neg	negative	_____
NIDDM, Type II	non-insulin dependent diabetes mellitus	_____
NPO	nothing by mouth	_____
OD	right eye (oculus dexter)	_____
OP	outpatient	_____
OR	operating room	_____
OREF	open reduction external fixation	_____
ORIF	open reduction internal fixation	_____
OS or OL	left eye (oculus sinister, oculus laevus)	_____
	both eyes (oculi unitas)	_____
OU	each eye (oculus uterque)	_____
P	pulse	_____
PA	posteroanterior	_____
pc	after meals (postcibum)	_____
PDR	*Physicians' Desk Reference*	_____
PERRLA	pupils equal, round, reactive to light and accommodation	_____
PI	present illness	_____
po	by mouth (per os)	_____
PO	postoperative	_____
pm	afternoon or evening (post meridiem)	_____
prn	as needed or desired (pro re nata)	_____
PSA	prostate specific antigen	_____
q	every (quaque)	_____
qh	every hour (quaque hora)	_____
q2h	every two hours	_____

qid	four times a day (quater in die)	_____
qm	every morning (quaque mane)	_____
qn	every night (quaque nocte)	_____
R	right, respiration	_____
RA	rheumatoid arthritis	_____
RBC	red blood cell, erythrocyte count	_____
Rh	blood factor, Rh+ or Rh−	_____
RLQ	right lower quadrant (abdomen)	_____
R/O	rule out	_____
RPh	registered pharmacist	_____
RUQ	right upper quadrant (abdomen)	_____
RVT	registered vascular technologist	_____
s̄, w/o	without (sine)	_____
sc, subcu, sq	subcutaneously (into fat layer)	_____
sed rate	sedimentation rate (erythrocyte)	_____
SOB	short of breath	_____
SOS	if necessary (si opus sit)	_____
s̄s̄, 1/2, .5	half (semis—Latin)	_____
staph	staphylococcus	_____
stat	immediately (statim)	_____
STI	sexually transmitted infection	_____
strep	streptococcus	_____
Sx	symptoms	_____
T1, T2, T3 . . . T12	thoracic vertebrae: first, second, third . . . twelfth	_____
T	temperature	_____

tab(s)	tablets	_____
TC&DB	turn, cough, and deep breathe	_____
Td	tetatnus toxoid	_____
tid	three times a day (ter in die)	_____
tinct	tincture	_____
TPN	total parenteral nutrition	_____
ULQ	upper left quadrant (abdomen)	_____
ung	ointment (unguentum)	_____
URQ	upper right quadrant (abdomen)	_____
Var	varicella (chickenpox) vaccine	_____
WBC	white blood cell, leukocyte count	_____
wm, bm	white male, black male	_____
wf, bf	white female, black female	_____
$\times$	times, power	_____
$-$	negative	_____
F, ♀	female	_____
M, ♂	male	_____
$\pm$	positive or negative	_____
*	birth	_____
†	death	_____
$\bar{p}$	after (post—Latin)	_____
$\bar{a}$	before (ante—Latin)	_____
#	pound, number	_____
↑	increase, above, elevated	_____
↓	decrease, below, lowered	_____
>	greater than	_____
<	less than	_____
°	degree, gallon, hour	_____

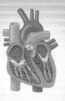

APPENDIX B
History and Physical Exam Report

CHIEF COMPLAINT: ABDOMINAL PAIN

SOURCE: PATIENT—RELIABLE

HISTORY OF PRESENT ILLNESS: The patient is a 70-year-old white male with diffuse **atherosclerotic** vascular disease, status **post** right carotid **endarterectomy,** and **aortic abdominal aneurysectomy** with repair and bypass and a **coronary artery bypass graft** times four in March 1997. On the day of admission, the patient developed a severe, sharp, persistent, constant, sometimes intermittently crampy abdominal pain in the **periumbilical** area, which radiated to the back and diffusely throughout the entire abdomen. The pain woke the patient from a sound sleep at 3:00 A.M. and became progressively worse throughout the day. The patient felt nauseated but did not vomit. He felt that if he could vomit, he would feel better. The patient denied any **diarrhea** or **constipation** but stated that his last bowel movement was very small and occurred in the morning on the day of admission. The patient denied any fever but felt hot with chills, and denied any sweating, cough, or shaking rigors. The patient stated that for lunch he had some soup and crackers. At 3:00 P.M. he had a small bowl of ice cream, after which the symptoms intensified tremendously. The patient called me and was directed to come to the emergency room.

PAST MEDICAL HISTORY: The patient denies a history of **diabetes mellitus** but admits to a history of **hypertension.** Denies any heart attack, **congestive heart failure, rheumatic** heart disease, **hepatitis, jaundice, hyperthyroidism,** rheumatic **valvular** heart disease, **hypothyroidism,** Addison's disease, or Cushing's disease. Surgical history included the abdominal aortic **aneurysm** repair and bypass, right carotid endarterectomy, four coronary artery bypass grafts, and facial surgery after an airplane accident in the mid 1960s. Medical hospitalizations: essentially none. Medications: patient is presently taking only Dyazide for control of blood pressure. Allergies: none; however, when the patient takes Dermerol, and is very sensitive to it, becoming very confused and disoriented.

SYSTEMIC REVIEW: The patient denies any shortness of breath, chest pain, **dyspnea** on exertion, cough, sputum production, **asthma, emphysema,** or **bronchitis.** No **palpitations, claudication,** irregular heartbeat, or **pedal** edema. GI: per history of the present illness. GU: no **dysuria, pyuria, hematuria,** increased frequency or urgency. No **arthralgia** or **myalgias.**

SOCIAL HISTORY: The patient lives with his wife. He does not smoke cigarettes, drink alcohol, or use any drugs.

PHYSICAL EXAMINATION

GENERAL: Reveals the patient to be in no acute distress. Temperature is 95.4°, pulse 82, blood pressure 138/82, respiratory rate 20.

HEAD AND NECK: HEENT: Grossly within normal limits. Neck: supple, full range of motion. No **jugular venous pressure distension,** no **thyromegaly,** lymph nodes, or masses. Scar over right neck from right carotid endarterectomy. Questionable slight **bruit** Grade I present over the right carotid; none present over the left.

SPINE: Benign, nontender. No **paravertebral** muscle spasm. No **costovertebral** angle tenderness.

CHEST AND HEART: Lungs are clear to **percussion** and **auscultation.** COR: regular rate and rhythm. Heart sounds are distant S1 and S2 **physiological.** No appreciable S3 and S4, murmur, or rub.

ABDOMEN: Slightly distended. Bowel sounds are present, tender in the **midepigastrium** and slightly in the **right upper quadrant** with mild **guarding.** No **rigidity,** no **rebound.**

GU AND RECTAL: Rectal examination reveals the **prostate** to be smooth without nodules. Stool is negative for **occult blood. Genitalia** reveals the patient to have normal adult genitalia. No appreciable **hernia. Testicles** are both descended without any masses appreciable.

EXTREMITIES: No **edema, cyanosis, clubbing.** Negative Homan's sign; negative for calf tenderness.

NEUROLOGICAL: The patient is alert and oriented. **Cranial** nerves II through XII are grossly within normal limits. **Ambulatory.** Moves all four extremities. Strength is **symmetrical.** Deep tendon reflexes are two plus and **symmetrical. Plantar reflexes** are downgoing.

IMPRESSION:

1. Acute abdomen with multiple dilated loops of small bowel. Mechanical bowel **obstruction** versus an **ileus.** Rule out **adhesions** secondary to **abdominal** surgery. Rule out **cholecystitis, diverticulitis,** and **pancreatitis.**

2. **Hypertension,** under control.

3. Diffuse **atherosclerotic vascular disease,** status post right carotid endarterectomy. Abdominal aortic aneurysm repair. Coronary artery bypass graft times four.

4. Arteriosclerotic coronary vascular disease, asymptomatic.

PLAN: Admit patient, **IV hydration, NPO,** follow serial laboratories, and obtain a surgical consult.

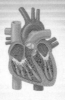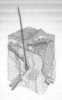

APPENDIX C
Glossary of Proper Noun Medical Terms

Addison's disease—deficiency in adrenocortical hormones caused by a progressive destruction of the adrenal glands.

Bartholin cyst—cyst of the gland located in the cleft between the labia minora and the hymenal ring that secretes mucous lubricant.

Bell's palsy—idiopathic facial palsy of CN VII resulting in asymmetry of the palpebral fissures, nasolabial folds, mouth, and facial expression on the affected side.

Biot's respirations—irregularly irregular respiratory pattern caused by damage to the medulla.

Bouchard's node—bony enlargement of the proximal interphalangeal joint of the finger.

Braxton Hicks contractions—uterine contractions that are irregular and painless; also known as false labor.

Brushfield's spots—small, white flecks located around the perimeter of the iris and associated with Down's syndrome.

Cesarean section—delivery of the fetus by abdominal surgery (hysterotomy).

Chadwick's sign—blue soft cervix occurring normally during pregnancy.

Chandelier's sign—cervix motion tenderness on palpation.

Cheyne-Stokes respirations—crescendo/decrescendo respiratory pattern interspersed between periods of apnea.

Cooley's anemia—thalassemia major.

Coombs' test—postnatal blood test of cord blood for antibodies against fetal blood type (Rh-negative mother, Rh-positive fetus).

Crohn's disease—regional ileitis; inflammatory bowel disease.

Cullen's sign—bluish color encircling the umbilicus and indicative of blood in the peritoneal cavity.

Cushing's syndrome—hypersecretion of the adrenal cortex causing excessive production of glucocorticoids; may be caused by a turmor.

Down's syndrome—extra chromosome (trisomy) of 21 or 22; variety of signs and symptoms, including retardation, flopping forehead, flat nose or absent bridge, and generally dwarfed physique.

Electra complex—girl's sexual attraction to her father and rivalry with her mother.

Fallopian tubes—uterine tubes.

Giardia—genus of protozoan flagellate causing dysentery.

Glasgow coma scale—international scale used in grading neurological response.

Graafian follicle—mature vesicular follicle of the ovary; matures ovum and secretes estrogen and progesterone.

Grave's disease—disease characterized by hyperthyroidism, exophthalmic goiter, and thyromegaly, and dermopathy.

Guillan-Barre syndrome—autoimmune inflammation causing destruction of the myelin sheath.

Harlequin color change—one-half of the newborn's body is red or ruddy and the other half appears pale.

Heberden's node—enlargement of the distal interphalangeal joint of the finger.

HELLP syndrome—pregnancy-induced hypertension, hemolysis, elevated liver enzymes and low platelets.

Hirsutism—excessive body hair.

Hodgkin's disease—cancerous lymphoreticular tumor.

Homan's sing—pain in the calf when the foot is dorsiflexed

Horner's syndrome—paralysis of the cervical sympathetic nerve causing contracted pupil and blepharoptosis.

Korotkoff sounds—sounds generated when the flow of blood through an artery is altered by the inflation of a blood pressure cuff around the extremity.

Korsakoff's syndrome—polyneuritic psychosis caused by chronic alcoholism.

Kussmaul's respirations—respirations characterized by extreme increased rate and depth, as in diabetic ketoacidosis.

Lou Gehrig's disease—amyotrophic lateral sclerosis.

Mantoux test—test for tuberculosis.

McBurney's point—anatomic location that is approximately at the normal location of the appendix in the RLQ; point of increased tenderness in appendicitis.

Mongolian spots—various irregularly sized areas of deep bluish pigmentation on the upper back, shoulders, buttocks, and lumbosacral area of newborn of African, Latino, and Asian decent.

Mongolism—obsolete term for Down's syndrome.

Montgomery's tubercles—sebaceous and milk glands present on the areola that produce secretions during breast-feeding.

Murphy's sing—abnormal finding elicited during abdominal palpation in the RUQ and revealing gallbladder inflammation; patient will abruptly stop inspiration and complain of a sharp pain.

Nabothian cysts—small, round, yellow lesions on the cervical surface.

Non-Hodgkin's lymphoma—lymphoma that arises directly from the thymus gland.

Oedipus complex—boy's sexual attraction to his mother and feelings of rivalry toward his father.

Paget's disease—(1) malignant neoplasm of the mammary ducts; (2) osteitis deformans.

Papanicolaou test—Pap smear; a tissue slide examination to detect cervical cancer.

Parkinson's disease—chronic degenerative nerve disease characterized by palsy, muscle stiffness and weakness, tremor, and fatigue and malaise.

Persian Gulf syndrome—variety of symptoms experienced by veterans of the Persian Gulf war, including respiratory, gastrointestinal, joint, and muscle discomforts, fatigue, and memory loss.

Rosving's sign—technique to elicit referred pain indicative of peritoneal inflammation.

Skene's glands—paraurethral glands.

Snellen chart—chart used for testing distance vision using standardized numbers and letters of various sizes.

Stensen's ducts—openings from the parotid glands.

Tay-Sachs disease—autosomal recessive trait, inherited, causing lack of hexosaminase A; this disease is characterized by mental and physical retardation, blindness, convulsions, cephalomegaly, and death by age 4.

Tourette's syndrome—symptoms include lack of muscle coordination, spasms, tics, grunts, barks, involuntary swearing, and coprolalia.

Weber's test—tuning fork used to measure hearing loss and determine if it is conductive or sensorineural.

Wharton's ducts—openings to the submaxillary glands.

References

Estes, *Health Assessment & Physical Examination*. Delmar, 1997.

Stedman's 27th edition. Lippincott & Williams & Wilkins, 1999.

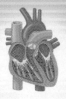 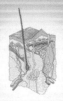

APPENDIX D
Additional Word Parts

Following are word parts in addition to those presented in the frames. Use these lists, your knowledge of word building, and your medical dictionary to enrich your medical vocabulary.

1. Pick a word part from the alphabetic list that interests you.

2. Look for it in your medical dictionary.

3. Find words that begin or end with this part and make a list.

4. Write the meanings of the new words you discovered.

5. Use the key in your dictionary to decipher the correct pronunciation and practice saying the new words

Word Part	Meaning	Example
acid/o	acid	acid/osis
acne	point	acne vulgaris
actin/o	ray (radiation)	actin/o/dermat/itis
acu	needle	acu/puncture
adenoid	resembling a gland	aden/oid/ectomy
adnex/al	adjacent, accessory	adnex/ectomy
albin/o	white	albin/ism
alkal/o	base	alkal/osis
all/o	other, different	all/o/pathy, all/ergy
ambly/o	dim, dull	ambly/opia
amyl/o	starch	amyl/ase
andr/o	man	andr/o/gen
aneurysm/o	abnormal dilation	aneurysm/o/rrhaphy
aort/o	aorta	aort/o/graphy
atel/o	imperfect, collapsed	atel/ectasis
bar/o	weight, heavy	bar/iatrics
bil/i	bile	bil/i/rubin

Word Part	Meaning	Example
cac/o	bad, diseased	cac/hexia
cat/a	down, downward	cat/a/tonic
celi/o	abdominal region	celi/ac artery
cerumin/o	wax	cerumin/o/lysis
chalas/ia	relaxation	a/chalas/ia
chem/o	chemical, drug	chem/o/therapy
chron/o	time	chronological, chronic
chym/o	juice	ec/chym/o/sis
cirrh/o	orange-yellow	cirrh/o/sis
-clasia	breaking down	arthr/o/clasia
-cleisis	closure, occlusion	colp/o/cleis/is
coll/o	glutinous, jellylike	coll/agen
cry/o	freezing	cry/o/surgery
decub/o	lying down	decubit/us ulcer
eczem/o	boil out	eczem/a
effer/	to bring out	effer/ent
effus/o	to pour out	effus/ion
fec/a	feces	fec/a/lith
glomerul/o	glomerulus	glomerul/o/nephr/itis
gonad/o	ovaries, testes	gonad/o/tropin
halit/o	breath	halit/o/sis
kal/i	potassium	hyper/kal/emia
kary/o	nucleus	kary/o/type
ket/o	ketones	ket/o/sis
klept/o	stealing	klept/o/mania
kyph/o	humped	kyph/o/sis
lord/o	bending	lord/o/sis
mediastin/o	mediastinum	mediastin/al
morph/o	form	meso/morph/ic
muscul/o	muscle	muscul/o/skelet/al
natr/i	sodium	hyper/natr/emia
-orexis	appetite	an/orex/ia
pach/y	thick	pach/y/dermat/ous
-poiesis	produce, form	hemat/o/poies/is
poikil/o	irregular shape	poikil/o/cyt/o/sis
prax/ia	action	a/prax/ia
prur/i	itch	prur/itus

Word Part	Meaning	Example
pteryg/o	wing	pteryg/o/mandibul/ar
ptyal/o	saliva	ptyal/in
radicul/o	root	radicul/o/neur/itis
roentgen/o	x-ray	roentgen/o/graphy
scoli/o	lateral curve	scoli/o/sis
scot/o	darkness	scot/oma
seb/o	fatty, sebum	seb/o/rrhea
sial/o	saliva	sial/aden/itis
somat/o	body	psych/o/somat/ic
sphygm/o	pulse	sphygm/o/man/o/meter
sphyx/o	pulse (related to O_2)	a/sphyxia
stere/o	solid, three-dimensional	stere/o/metry
steth/o	chest	steth/o/scope
-sthenia	strength	my/e/sthen/ia
stigmat/o	mark, point	a/stigmat/ism
taxia	muscle coordination	a/tax/ia
tel/e	distant, far	tel/e/metry
terat/o	monster, wonder	terat/o/genic
tetra	four	tetra/cycline
thel/o	nipple	thel/o/rrhagia
tresia	perforation, closure	a/tres/ia
vagin/o	vagina	vagin/itis
varic/o	twisted vein	varic/o/sity
vulv/o	vulva	vulv/o/vagin/itis
xen/o	strange, foreign	xen/o/phob/ia
xer/o	dry	xer/o/derma

Source: Smith, Davis, Dennerll, *Medical Technology: A programmed systems approach,* 8th ed.

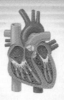 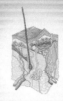

APPENDIX E
Answers to Review Exercises

Word-Building System Review Answers

1. a   2. d   3. a   4. d   5. d   6. c   7. b   8. d   9. a   10. b

Practicing Plurals:

1. bacilli
2. diagnoses
3. cervices
4. ganglia
5. ilia
6. lipomata

Transforming Nouns to Adjectives:

1. cyanotic
2. anemic
3. carpal
4. iliac

UNIT 1 REVIEW EXERCISE ANSWERS
Part 2:

1. h
2. d
3. i
4. m
5. f
6. a
7. l
8. n
9. j
10. b

Part 3:

1. acrodermatitis
2. posterior, back
3. inferior
4. lateral
5. thoracic
6. proximal
7. pleural
8. dermatopathy (dermopathy)
9. acromegaly
10. dermatologist

Part 4:
1. cells
2. cytology, histologist
3. etiology, dermatitis
4. distal
5. mucosa
6. serous

7. pericardium

8. pelvic, inferior

9. anterior

10. lateral

Part 5:

1. anatomy and physiology

2. hydrochloric acid

3. left lower quadrant

4. right upper quadrant

5. anteroposterior

6. posteroanterior

7. right lower quadrant

Part 6:

1. cephalic
2. hyper, super, supra, superior
3. hypo, sub, inferior
4. antero, ventro,
   anterior, ventral
5. circum

6. poster/o, dors/o,
   posterior, ventral
7. lateral
8. medial
9. distal, dist/o
10. proximal, proxim/o

UNIT 2 REVIEW EXERCISE SELF TEST ANSWERS

Part 2:

1. i	5. m	8. e
2. a	6. b	9. f
3. h	7. j	10. d
4. l		

Part 3:

1. echocardiography	5. thrombophlebitis	8. hemolysis
2. cardialgia	6. thrombogenic	9. hemangioma
3. tachycardia	7. lymphoma	10. angiopathy
4. arteriosclerosis		

Part 4:

1. leukoderma, melanocytes	5. thrombocytes	9. radiographer
2. leukocytopenia, leukocytosis	6. thrombus	10. tachycardia
3. ischemic	7. cardiologist	
4. cytolysis	8. sonography	

Part 5:

1. CABG	coronary artery bypass graft
2. Diff	WBC differential
3. HGB	hemoglobin
4. AMI	acute myocardial infarction
5. TIA	transient ischemic attack
6. XR	radiogram
7. CBC	complete blood count
8. HCT	hematocrit
9. AA	aortic aneurysm
10. PVC	premature ventricular contraction

UNIT 3 EXERCISE ACTIVITY ANSWERS

Part 2:

1. d	5. h	8. j
2. g	6. f	9. o
3. k	7. a	10. l
4. n		

Part 3:

1. adenitis	5. oncologist	8. lipoid
2. melanocarcinoma	6. visceral	9. cranioplasty
3. adenectomy	7. antineoplastic	
4. neurology		

Part 4:

1. neurologist	4. leiomyoma	7. hypertrophy
2. myelocele	5. cephalic	8. melanocytes
3. histolysis	6. neophobia	9. psychiatrist

Part 5:

1. Ca	cancer
2. RT(T)	radiologic technician (radiation therapy)
3. metas	metastasis
4. EEG	electroencephalogram
5. ASCP	American Society of Clinical Pathology

6. CNS   central nervous system

7. IPV   inactivated polis vaccine

UNIT 4 EXERCISE ACTIVITY ANSWERS

Part 2:

1. o	5. p	8. k
2. f	6. b	9. c
3. h	7. n	10. i
4. l		

Part 3:

1. abdominocentesis	6. gastroenteric (gastrointestinal)
2. enteroscope	7. cholecystogram
3. gastroduodenostomy	8. pancreatolith
4. dysphagia	9. neurotripsy
5. splenomegaly	10. malnutrition

Part 4:

1. cholecystogram	5. malnutrition
2. gastrorrhagia, peptic	6. amniocentesis
3. dysentery	7. sublingually
4. tachyphagia	8. gingivitis

Part 5:

1. PC	after meals	6. EGD	esophagogastro-duodenoscopy
2. ERCP	endoscopic retrograde cholangiopancreatography	7. GB	gallbladder
3. HAA	hepatitis associated antigen		
4. BM	bowel movement		
5. NPO	nothing by mouth		

UNIT 5 EXERCISE ACTIVITY ANSWERS

Part 2:

1. Ca^{++}	calcium ion
2. CPD	cephalopelvic disproportion
3. C_2	second cervical vertebra
4. OA	osteoarthritis

5. DO   doctor of osteopathy

6. Fx   fracture

7. DDS   dentist

8. ORTH   orthopedist

Part 3:

1. f   6. k

2. d   7. m

3. h   8. o

4. g   9. a

5. l   10. n

Part 4:

1. acromioclavicular   6. thoracocentesis

2. epicondyle   7. humer/o

3. sacroiliac   8. kinesiology

4. metacarpals   9. osteoporosis

5. myofibroma   10. orthodontist

Part 5:

1. phalanx, ischium   5. carpal

2. tendonitis   6. diskectomy, laminectomy

3. arthritis, arthroscope   7. FxBB, radioulnar

4. pelvimetry

UNIT 6 REVIEW EXERCISE ANSWERS

Part 2:

1. o   6. k

2. f   7. j

3. g   8. c

4. l   9. a

5. m   10. n

Part 3:

1. urethritis   3. nocturia, nycturia

2. cystorrhagia   4. nephropyelitis

5. vasodilation, vasodilatation

6. ureterorrhaphy

7. orchiocele, orchidocele

8. nephroptosis

9. incontinence

10. dehydration

Part 4:

1. urologist, testicular

2. prostatic, BPH

3. pyelogram, ureterolith

4. dehydrated

5. incision, excise

6. cystorrhagia

7. hydrophobia

8. vasectomy

Part 5:

1. ESRD	end stage renal disease
2. KUB	kidney, ureter, bladder x-ray
3. PKU	phenylketonuria
4. UTI	urinary tract infection
5. M, ♂	male
6. Cysto	cystoscopy
7. IVP	intravenous pyelogram
8. BUN	blood urea nitrogen

UNIT 7 REVIEW EXERCISE ANSWERS

Part 2:

1. f

2. m

3. l

4. n

5. o

6. c

7. k

8. b

9. d

10. e

Part 3:

1. mastocarcinoma

2. mammogram (mammograph)

3. anisocytosis

4. prenatal (antenatal)

5. gynecologist

6. primigravida

7. nullipara (nulliparous)

8. syphilophobia

9. mammography

10. ectopic

Part 4:

1. multigravida, aborted, bipara

2. anisomastia, mammoplasty

3. endometriosis

4. hysteroscope

5. syphilopsychosis

6. ovum, ovulation

Part 5:

1. D&C	dilation and curettage	5. Pap	Papanicolaou test
2. FTT	failure to thrive	6. PMS	premenstrual syndrome
3. OB	obstetrics	7. F, ♀	female
4. HSG	hysterosalpingogram	8. Para 1	one viable birth

UNIT 8 REVIEW EXERCISE ANSWERS

Part 2:

1. tympanotomy (myringotomy)

2. nasopharyngitis

3. aphasia

4. audiometer

5. lacrimation

6. nyctalopia

7. iridocele

8. blepharitis

9. ophthalmoscope

10. hyperopia

Part 3:

1. l

2. r

3. q

4. k

5. i

6. j

7. g

8. m

9. a

10. n

Part 4:

1. nyctalopia

2. diaphragm, diaphragm

3. pulmonary

4. pneumothorax, anisocoria

5. audiologist, myopia, keratotomy

6. aphasia

7. endotracheal

Part 5:

1. LA	light and accommodation
2. OD	right eye
3. AS	left ear
4. TB	tuberculosis
5. OS	left eye
6. ENT	otorhinolaryngologist
7. COPD	chronic obstructive pulmonary disease
8. URI	upper respiratory infection

UNIT 9 REVIEW EXERCISE ANSWERS

Part 2:

1. adhesions	6. microscope
2. abduction	7. homosexual
3. circumduction	8. heterogeneous
4. perforate	9. congenital
5. dissect	10. injection

Part 3:

1. h	6. p
2. l	7. m
3. k	8. q
4. i	9. g
5. d	10. n

Part 4:

1. transposition	6. heterosexual
2. ultraviolet	7. pericardium
3. contraindicated	8. macrocyte
4. superficial	9. retroversion
5. homolateral	10. adduction

UNIT 10 REVIEW EXERCISE ANSWERS

Part 2:

1. o	6. d
2. g	7. m
3. k	8. p
4. i	9. l
5. q	10. a

Part 3:

1. synergistic	6. malaria
2. sympodia	7. hyperthyroidism
3. adrenomegaly	8. testosterone
4. prognosis	9. endocrinologist
5. prodromal	10. otorhinolaryngologist

Part 4:

1. dietitian, insulin, endocrinologist
2. dermatologist, biopsy
3. syndrome, septicemia
4. neurologist, diagnosis, prognosis
5. immunity, immunodeficiency syndrome

Part 5:

1. Bx	biopsy	6. IPV	inactivated polio vaccine
2. Rx	prescribe	7. Hx	history
3. Tx	treatment	8. TSH	thyroid stimulating hormone
4. Dx	diagnosis	9. MMRV	measles, mumps, rubella vaccine
5. SIDS	sudden infant death syndrome	10. HPV	human papillomavirus

Part 6:

1. pituitary gland	5. testis
2. thymus gland	6. adrenal gland
3. pancreas (islets of Langerhans)	7. thyroid gland
4. ovary	8. pineal gland

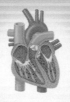
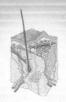

APPENDIX F
Crossword Puzzle Solutions

Unit 1 Puzzle

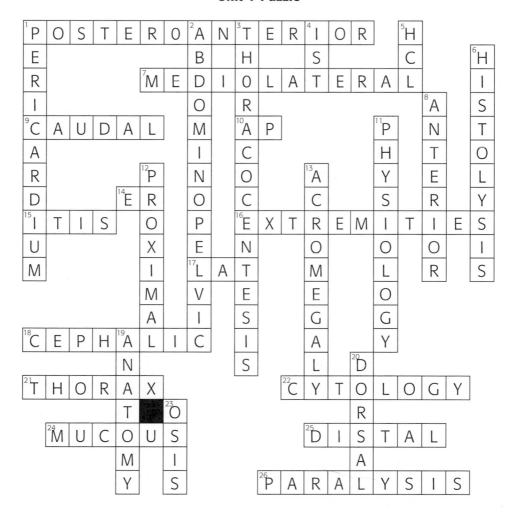

Unit 2 Puzzle

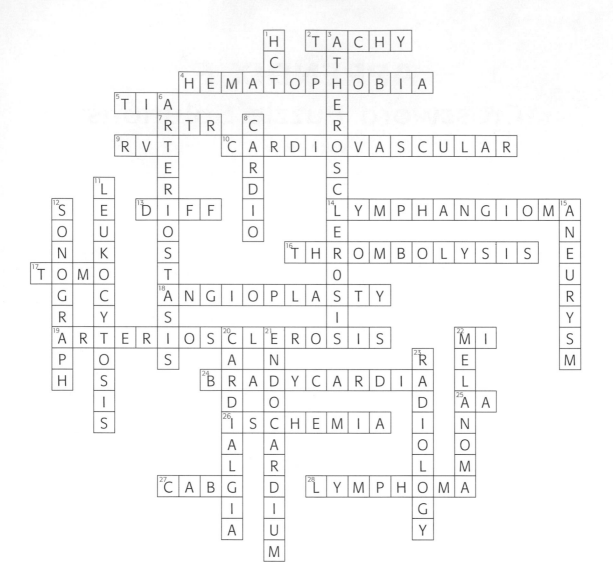

Unit 3 Puzzle

Crossword puzzle with the following filled answers:

- MUCOID
- ELECTROENCEPHALOGRAPH
- CEREBROVASCULAR
- ENCEPHALOPATHY
- MUCORANIN (vertical: ARANI...)
- HYPERTROPHY
- RTR
- CELIAL
- MENINGOCELE
- SARCOMA
- EEG
- ENCEPHALOCELE
- MELANOCYTE
- NEUROLOGIST
- ATHEROSCLEROSIS
- HYDROLOGIST
- CRANIOTOMY
- MENINGIA
- NEUROSURGEON
- HYPERPLASIA
- CEREBRITIS
- DYSPLASIA
- HISTOLOGY
- CARCINOMA
- NEUROLYSIS
- STROMA
- ONCOLOGIST
- VISCERAL
- MALIGNANT
- NEOPLASM
- LIPOMA
- MUCOUS
- PARIETAL
- MYELITIS

Unit 4 Puzzle

Across and down entries:

- SUBGLOSSAL
- MALNUTRITION
- DIVERTICULA
- SPLENIC
- GINGIVITIS
- STOMATALGIA
- PANCREATOLITH
- RECTOCELE
- COLON
- TACHY
- HEPATO
- ULCER
- RRHAPHY
- MALAISE
- DYSPEPSIA
- TRICHO
- RRHEA
- ABDOMINOCENTESIS
- ABDOMINO

Down letters:
- MA / MALPO
- CHOLECYSTPTSIS (CHOLECYSTPTSIS column: C H O L E C Y S T P T S I S)
- BRADYPHGIA column letters
- SCALP column
- SUBLINGUA column
- GASTRSTOMY column
- ESTPGEA column
- PHGIAA column
- SHAGG column
- CUPPOTIO column
- ENTERITI column
- HEMORRHOI column
- ECYSTECTO column
- RRHAGE column
- HBY column
- DIETITI column
- AN column
- B column

Unit 5 Puzzle

A completed crossword puzzle with the following answers:

Across:
- 1. KINESIOLOGY
- 5. ARTHROPLASTY
- 7. DOR
- 9. THORACIC
- 10. CALCANEUS
- 12. ORTHODONTIST
- 14. ARTHROSCOPY
- 17. FEMORO
- 21. TIBIA
- 22. METATARSALS
- 23. OSTEOARTHROPATHY
- 24. PUBIS
- 26. FEMUR
- 29. PELVIMETRY
- 31. EPICONDYLE
- 36. ACROMION
- 37. XIPHOID
- 38. MYOPATHY
- 39. MALACIA
- 40. DENTOID

Down:
- 2. OSTEP
- 3. THORACO
- 4. DECALCIFICATION
- 6. RHEEMATA
- 8. INTERPROR
- 11. TENDONITIS
- 13. RADIOULNAR
- 15. ARTHROSIS
- 16. HYPERTROPHY
- 18. ISCHIRDRI
- 19. ATROPOPD
- 20. COSTOSCOPHY
- 25. PHALANAN
- 27. TIBION
- 28. MYOG
- 30. CERVICAL
- 32. LIGAMENTS
- 33. CRAPPLYS
- 34. COCCYX
- 35. SUR

Unit 6 Puzzle

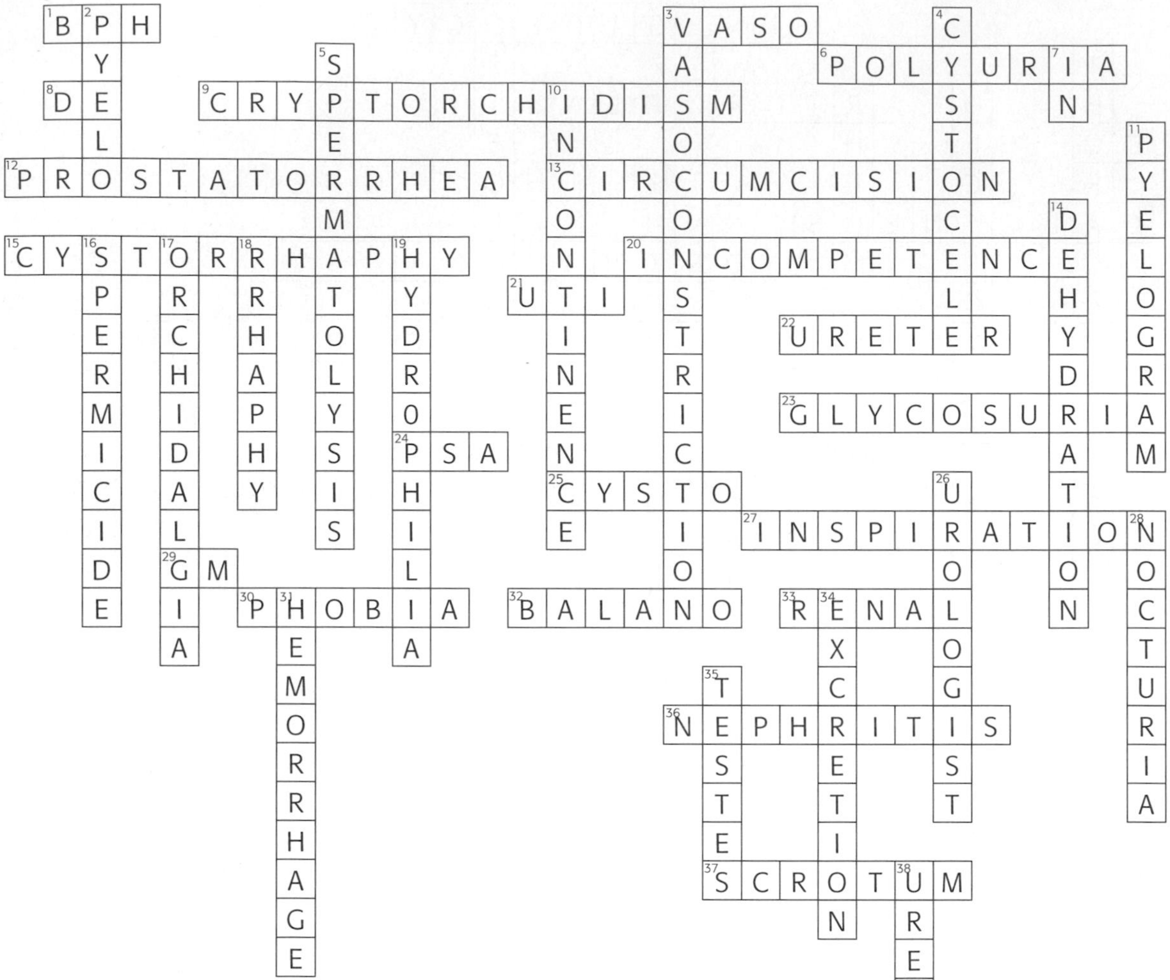
1 BPH
2 PYELO
3 VASO
3 VASOCONSTRICTIO
4 CYSTOCELE
5 SPERMATOLYSIS
6 POLYURIA
7 IN
8 DE
9 CRYPTORCHIDISM
10 INCONTINENCE
11 PYELOGRAM
12 PROSTATORRHEA
13 CIRCUMCISION
14 DEHYDRATION
15 CYSTORRHAPHY
16 SPERMICIDE
17 ORCHIDALGIA
18 RRHAPHY
19 HYDR0PHILIA
20 INCOMPETENCE
21 UTI
22 URETER
23 GLYCOSURIA
24 PSA
25 CYSTO
26 UROLOGIST
27 INSPIRATION
28 NOCTURIA
29 GM
30 PHOBIA
31 HEMORRHAGE
32 BALANO
33 RENAL
34 EXCRETION
35 TESTE
36 NEPHRITIS
37 SCROTUM
38 URETHRA

Unit 7 Puzzle

1 SYPHILOPATHY 4 H(YS) 5 ANTE 7 M
8 M 2 OB 3 AB 4 HYS 6 END 9 HY
10 SALPINGITIS 11 HYSTEROPTOSIS 13 HSG
14 C 17 DYSMENORRHEA
15 NEONATAL 16 OB 18 S
19 FTT
20 GYNECOLOGIST 21 ISO
22 LAPAROTOMY
23 MAMMOGRAPHY
25 B
26 INFRAMAMMARY 27 CERVICAL
28 LAPAROSCOPY 29 P 30 R
31 OVULATION
32 NULLIPAROUS 33 P 34 O 35 PRENATAL 36 A
37 I
38 MULTIPARA 39 A

Unit 8 Puzzle

Crossword puzzle grid with the following answers:

1. PRESBYOPIA
2. OPHTHALMITIS
3. SQUINT
4. NASOSCOPE
5. PHCORNEMEM (vertical PH...)
6. BLEPHARITIS
7. OPTOMETER
8. URI
9. RETINOPLASTY
10. PLACCEME
11. NYCTALO
12. PNEUMONOMELANOSIS
13. LPHTHALMGOPLF
14. O
15. DYS
16. ASTHMA
17. OTT
18. PNEUMO
19. OPTIC
20. CORNEOSCLERAL
21. EMLLM
22. I
23. KELAST
24. RHINOPLASTY
25. LARYNG
26. BRONCHORRHAGIA
27. PHPHCHHL
28. ADECTOMY
29. TYPY
30. AUDIO
31. PNEUMONITIS
32. PERTUSSIS
33. ENDOTRACHEAL
34. THORAX
35. AMBI
36. AUDIOLOGY
37. TRACHEOSTOMY
38. PHARYX
39. LACRIMAL
40. ESOTROPIA
41. HEENT
42. OTALGIA
43. DYSPHONIA
44. RRHEA
45. APNEA
46. LARYNGES

Unit 9 Puzzle

Across:

4. EXTRA-ARTICULAR
6. PERIODONTAL
8. SINISTROMANUAL
11. METASTASIZE
13. INTRAUTERINE
15. SEMICONSCIOUS
20. RETRO
21. SUPRAINGUINAL
23. CON
24. CONTRACEPTIVE
25. INTRACRANIAL
27. TRANSPOSITION
29. MICROCEPHALUS
32. TRANSVAGINAL
33. DEXTROCARDIA
34. HOMOLATERAL
36. PARACYSTITIS
39. HEMIPLEGIA
41. PO
42. PERCUTANEOUS
43. PODIATRIST
44. HETEROSEXUAL
45. INTER
46. ADDICTION
47. EFFUSION

Down:

1. EPIIO
2. AIS
3. INTR
5. CONTRABAND
7. O
9. ANTERE... (ANTERIOR)
10. HMMI
12. SUPERFICI...
14. CIRCUMDUCT...
17. IVERSION
18. CHIROPOD...
19. CIRCUMCI...
22. IM
25. INVERSION
26. ACTIN...
28. METACTOR
30. ULTR...
31. VERT...
35. ABDICATION
37. INJECTION
38. INSOMNIA
40. MAAL

Unit 10 Puzzle

1. HYPOTHYROIDISM
4. IDDM
8. IPV
10. ANTICONVULSIVE
11. DPM
16. THYROIDETCOMY
19. TESTOSTERONE
21. HYPERGLYCEMIA
23. ANTI
25. ENDOCRINOLOGIST
29. SYNDROME
33. EPINEPHRINE
35. MALARIA
36. HIV
37. VAR
39. CORTISONE
40. PHARMACIST

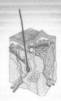

Index

Note: Indexing is by unit and frame number.

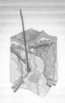

Index
of Word Parts
Learned

Note: Index is by unit and frame number.

System Requirements

Basic system requirements are:
- Microsoft® Windows® or better
- Pentium Processor
- Windows® Media Player® or comparable
- Double-spin CD-ROM drive

Set-Up Instructions

Computer CD

1. Insert the disk into the CD ROM player of your computer
2. The media player should automatically start up, and bring up track one

3. Use the media player as directed by the manufacturer (see its Help instructions for more information)

Audio CD

1. Insert the disk into the CD ROM player
2. The CD player should automatically start up, and bring up track one
3. Use the CD player as directed by the manufacturer

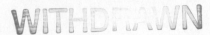

License Agreement for Delmar Learning, a division of Thomson Learning, Inc.

Educational Software/Data

You the customer, and Delmar Learning, a division of Thomson Learning, Inc. incur certain benefits, rights, and obligations to each other when you open this package and use the software/data it contains. BE SURE YOU READ THE LICENSE AGREEMENT CAREFULLY, SINCE BY USING THE SOFTWARE/DATA YOU INDICATE YOU HAVE READ, UNDERSTOOD, AND ACCEPTED THE TERMS OF THIS AGREEMENT.

Your rights:

1. You enjoy a non-exclusive license to use the software/data on a single microcomputer in consideration for payment of the required license fee, (which may be included in the purchase price of an accompanying print component), or receipt of this software/data, and your acceptance of the terms and conditions of this agreement.

2. You acknowledge that you do not own the aforesaid software/data. You also acknowledge that the software/data is furnished "as is," and contains copyrighted and/or proprietary and confidential information of Delmar Learning, a division of Thomson Learning, Inc. or its licensors.

There are limitations on your rights:

1. You may not copy or print the software/data for any reason whatsoever, except to install it on a hard drive on a single microcomputer and to make one archival copy, unless copying or printing is expressly permitted in writing or statements recorded on the diskette(s).

2. You may not revise, translate, convert, disassemble or otherwise reverse engineer the software/data except that you may add to or rearrange any data recorded on the media as part of the normal use of the software/data.

3. You may not sell, license, lease, rent, loan, or otherwise distribute or network the software/data except that you may give the software/data to a student or and instructor for use at school or, temporarily at home.

Should you fail to abide by the Copyright Law of the United States as it applies to this software/data your license to use it will become invalid. You agree to erase or otherwise destroy the software/data immediately after receiving note of termination of this agreement for violation of its provisions from Delmar Learning.

Delmar Learning, a division of Thomson Learning, Inc. gives you a LIMITED WARRANTY covering the enclosed software/data. The LIMITED WARRANTY follows this License.

This license is the entire agreement between you and Delmar Learning, a division of Thomson Learning, Inc. interpreted and enforced under New York law.

This warranty does not extend to the software or information recorded on the media. The software and information are provided "AS IS." Any

statements made about the utility of the software or information are not to be considered as express or implied warranties. Delmar Learning, a division of Thomson Learning, Inc. will not be liable for incidental or consequential damages of any kind incurred by you, the consumer, or any other user.

Some states do not allow the exclusion or limitation of incidental or consequential damages, or limitations on the duration of implied warranties so the above limitation or exclusion may not apply to you. This warranty gives you specific legal rights, and you may also have other rights which vary from state to state. Address all correspondence to: Delmar Learning, a division of Thomson Learning, Inc., 5 Maxwell Drive, P.O. Box 8007, Clifton Park, NY 12065-8007 Attention: Technology Department.

LIMITED WARRANTY

Delmar Learning, a division of Thomson Learning, Inc. warrants to the original licensee/purchaser of this copy of microcomputer software/ data and the media on which it is recorded that the media will be free from defects in material and workmanship for ninety (90) days from the date of original purchase. All implied warranties are limited in duration to this ninety (90) day period. THEREAFTER, ANY IMPLIED WARRANTIES, INCLUDING IMPLIED WARRANTIES OF MERCHANTABILITY AND FITNESS FOR A PARTICULAR PURPOSE, ARE EXCLUDED. THIS WARRANTY IS IN LIEU OF ALL OTHER WARRANTIES, WHETHER ORAL OR WRITTEN, EXPRESS OR IMPLIED.

If you believe the media is defective please return it during the ninety day period to the address shown below. Defective media will be replaced without charge provided that it has not been subjected to misuse or damage.

This warranty does not extend to the software or information recorded on the media. The software and information are provided "AS IS." Any statements made about the utility of the software or information are not to be considered as express or implied warranties.

Limitation of liability: Our liability to you for any losses shall be limited to direct damages, and shall not exceed the amount you paid for the software. In no event will we be liable to you for any indirect, special, incidental, or consequential damages (including loss of profits) even if we have been advised of the possibility of such damages.

Some states do not allow the exclusion or limitation of incidental or consequential damages, or limitations on the duration of implied warranties, so the above limitation or exclusion may not apply to you. This warranty gives you specific legal rights, and you may also have other rights which vary from state to state. Address all correspondence to: Delmar Learning, a division of Thomson Learning, Inc., 5 Maxwell Drive, P.O. Box 8007, Clifton Park, NY 12065-8007. Attention: Technology Department.